Trends in Language Acquisition Research

ISSN 1569-0644

TiLAR publishes monographs, edited volumes and text books on theoretical and methodological issues in the field of child language research. The focus of the series is on original research on all aspects of the scientific study of language behavior in children, linking different areas of research including linguistics, psychology & cognitive science.

For an overview of all books published in this series, please see
benjamins.com/catalog/tilar

Volume 25

Understanding Deafness, Language and Cognitive Development
Essays in honour of Bencie Woll
Edited by Gary Morgan

Understanding Deafness, Language and Cognitive Development

Essays in honour of Bencie Woll

Edited by

Gary Morgan
City University London

John Benjamins Publishing Company

Amsterdam / Philadelphia

The paper used in this publication meets the minimum requirements of the American National Standard for Information Sciences – Permanence of Paper for Printed Library Materials, ANSI z39.48-1984.

DOI 10.1075/tilar.25

Cataloging-in-Publication Data available from Library of Congress:
LCCN 2019036912 (PRINT) / 2019036913 (E-BOOK)

ISBN 978 90 272 0449 3 (HB)
ISBN 978 90 272 6186 1 (E-BOOK)

John Benjamins Publishing Company · www.benjamins.com

Table of contents

Foreword

Jim Kyle

Although the influence of the work of Bencie Woll expanded enormously with the creation of the Deafness Cognition and Language Centre (DCAL) at University College London, the roots of her involvement and commitment to the field of Deaf Studies and in particular early language development, can be seen in the work begun in the mid-1970s. As a new postgraduate, she joined Gordon Wells' language development project team in Bristol. The experience she gained in this work almost certainly shaped her whole outlook on the study of natural language development (some outcomes highlighted in Wells, 1981). When a different sort of challenge arose in Bristol in the first funded UK project on sign language, in 1978, she brought with her the skills in working on the complexities of spontaneous child language.

What follows in this section is a personal retrospective analysis which focuses on Bencie's contribution to the embryonic stage of a new discipline. Her work on deaf babies and children, begun in 1982, created a corpus which is still of value today, setting her on a pathway for research in the early acquisition of sign language, and in parallel produced the initial descriptions of British Sign Language (BSL).

The aim here is to consider the roots of this 'discipline' and to explore its origins from the 1970s in the UK. It is primarily a historical reflection and, to a degree, a case study of the significance of one person's role in that development. Other sections in this book deal with the expanding current literature dealing with deaf children and adults, their language and performance.

The thread for this reflection is the "Bristol Years and the Centre for Deaf Studies" and the key actor in this development is Bencie Woll, to whom this collection is dedicated. Some of the material is taken from the archives of the Centre for Deaf Studies in Bristol and may draw on internal reports and other professional interactions which are less well known. However, these are very important in understanding the early development of sign language research in the UK. These papers, which may not have been published externally, are available at <www.deafstudiestrust.org/cds-papers> or in the resources of the University of Bristol Library.

https://doi.org/10.1075/tilar.25.for
© 2020 John Benjamins Publishing Company

By 1978, the world of UK deaf education was changing (see also Tang, Adam & and Simpson, this volume). Various past attempts to assert the importance of sign language throughout the 20th century had proved to be unsuccessful and even the UK Government-commissioned report in 1968 in the UK on the potential role of fingerspelling in deaf schools (Lewis, 1968) failed to make an impact on teacher training and consequent classroom methodology. We were deep in an oralist phase of the treatment of deaf children and adults. This phase was characterised by faith in Audiology (which was combined with teacher training for deaf educa-tion), an approach that radiated from the University of Manchester, where the use of sign language was absent in the teacher training programme. Lack of central regulation by the UK Government (who suggested that each school was separately responsible for policies on language use for deaf children) and the almost com-plete absence of deaf teachers in the fifty schools for deaf children, produced a lack of debate on the national poor levels of achievement of deaf children. The cause of that failure of educational policy and practice was typically displaced to the deaf children and their families. 'Because they did not hear ...', 'because they did not use their hearing aids effectively ...' and even 'because their parents had not been strict enough in enforcing the speech only principles' were all beliefs shared throughout the teaching profession at that time. The term 'oral failure' was one of the most common descriptors for deaf young people who were members of the deaf community.

At the same time, maybe even paradoxically, deaf clubs were thriving. These local associations which existed in almost every town in the UK, catered for the regular meetings of a community ranging from deaf children, young adults right through to elderly people. They also supported a variety of activities – British Deaf Sports being particularly significant – and were the focal point of community life. This was where deaf people married, brought their children (hearing and deaf) and lived their lives.

It was probably three factors which came together to open the door to sign language research:

1. the general educational shift from the discourse of handicap and loss to a new idea of rights and special needs;
2. the undeniable and increasing evidence that deaf education was failing deaf pupils, and;
3. the advent of the video recording technology which could capture the com-munication of deaf people.

The latter, in particular, was a major catalyst, especially drawing linguists into the field. Their enthusiasm in examining and documenting the signs of deaf people led to the realisation and then the published claims that what deaf people did, was in fact, a language (see Deuchar, 1978).

The challenge had been and continued to be enormous for the Deaf community. Although there are records dating back over thousands of years that Deaf people existed, came together in communities and used a form of communication which involved the hands rather than the voice, they faced enormous obstacles in gaining acceptance in society.

In the UK, in the 1970s, deaf children were diagnosed late, provided with hearing aids, deterred in school from the use of the hands instead of the voice and were proactively offered community life by the missionary gatekeepers, who might also act as employment agents to place deaf people with local companies. Somehow the deaf community survived, socio-economically downwardly mobile, usually, but energetic in creating its own language and culture – the deaf way. The interest of linguists, at first treated with curiosity and then suspicion, came to be the stimulus for promotion and public awareness of the deaf voice.

Although there were advances in the USA and in particular, Stokoe's work on sign language (Stokoe, 1960),[1] this had not even by the mid-1970s created the momentum necessary for the coherent development of sign language research.

In 1978, there was no sign in BSL for the English word "language". In fact, older deaf people were resistant to the notion, having been told repeatedly that what they did with their hands was jumbled, incoherent and inadequate gesturing. "Language" was an English word to describe what hearing people did with their mouths. The notion that *language* included what deaf people made use of to exchange information and to express feelings was not understood even within the deaf community nor even among those whose parents were deaf (who would often advise their deaf children not to sign in public).

In 1978, the interest in sign language was mainly in its relation to systems which could support the need to display English visually. Signed English was promoted as the way forward in USA and in Sweden (Signed Swedish). These quickly ran into problems as signs did not map precisely on to words and were notably limited in extent of lexicon. This necessitated the introduction of artificial signs in order to be able to sign and speak at the same time (Evans, 1982, discussed the principles of combining signing and speaking).

There were very few voices if any, to challenge the public view that what deaf people did and what they termed "signing" was no more than a collection of gestures which could easily be learned by hearing people over a weekend (Dale, 1974) or what one influential social worker "for the deaf" termed the "secret language of

---

1. We could go even further back to 1874 with Tylor's description of sign language or even Scott's work from an educational point of view in 1870 to see where the origins lie in the UK.

the deaf." In the UK, a position paper by Mary Brennan presented to the British Deaf Association in 1974 (published 1976) and research by Margaret Deuchar (1978) based on recordings of interaction in Reading Deaf Club, near London, were all that was on offer to researchers. When Conrad (1979) surveyed all the schools in England and Wales, there was not a single school (of the 50 or so which operated) nor a single Unit in mainstream school which admitted to using sign language or even drew on a sign vocabulary. UK research began with two funded projects: one in Edinburgh led by Mary Brennan and one in Bristol, which Bencie Woll joined in late 1978. The work of the latter project evolved from an attempt to assess and train interpreters, to a focus on the newly discovered language.

The project summary indicated the aims of the three-year workplan to examine:

1. "the process involved in the use of sign language …
2. the characteristics of those who become effective communicators …
3. the communication powers of sign language through a linguistic study of British Sign Language as used by deaf people
4. … provision of signing instruction for interpreters, teachers, parents …

Two significant conferences followed from the quarterly meetings of the "sign language workshop": in 1980 (national, Woll, Kyle and Deuchar, 1981) and 1981 (international, Kyle and Woll, 1983).

We can describe the progress in in sign language research under four headings in regard to the impact of the work of Bencie Woll.

1. the discovery of British Sign Language to 1981 – promotion of BSL and its relevance to education and to community life.
2. consolidation of research to 1985 – the linguistic analysis in terms of phonology, syntax and pragmatics.
3. the examination of the acquisition of sign language – the recording and analysis of the emergence of sign language in deaf and hearing children in deaf families.
4. the comparison of different sign languages – international collection of sign languages based on the same lexicon and narrative texts.

All of these topics are particularly significant as foundations for the establishment of Deaf Studies in the UK, and her work on the linguistics of sign language is represented in a large number of publications on British Sign Language from 1979 onwards; however, only the third topic is explored here as being the most relevant to the theme of this book.

It was perhaps inevitable that having established the significance of sign language from a linguistic perspective that attention came to be focused on the analysis of BSL acquisition, given the very active research group in Bristol, sharing the same building as the sign language group. Gordon Well's contribution to child language work in the 1970s was to emphasise the need to obtain natural language recordings in home settings and to describe the interaction between child and caregiver, which led to mastery of that language (Wells, 1981). In 1982, fortuitously, and surprisingly, there were several deaf mothers expecting babies at almost the same time and permission was gained to record their babies' development from the age of three months. Thus began the detailed work on the emergence of sign language in deaf families (with both deaf and hearing children), which created a large and still extant database of recordings that was only completed with the publication of a final report to the research council in 2004 (see also the contributions of Harris & Clibbens and of Baker & van den Bogaerde, this volume for more extended analysis of this topic).

Work in Italy and the USA had already begun on early sign development by the time of the 1981 symposium. In Bristol recordings began in 1982, monthly at home and in the lab (from the age of 3 months) with 5 deaf children with deaf parents, 5 hearing children with deaf parents and for the first year, 8 hearing infants with hearing parents. Deaf children were added to the group as and when they were discovered. The data set had to move at the pace of the development of the children and so it was not until 1988 and 1989 that analysis could be appropriately reported. The Gesture to Sign and Speech final report (Kyle, Woll and Ackerman, 1989) to the Economic and Social Research Council sets out the detail of the methodology. Joint papers tackled lexical acquisition (Ackerman, Kyle, Woll and Ezra, 1990) and set out principles for the measurement of sign language development in deaf school children (Kirk, Kyle, Ackerman and Woll, 1990).

Although there are new insights and considerably expanded research work reported in later chapters in this book, it remains within the historic remit here to describe the beginnings of this work and to consider the analysis produced at this earlier time.

The first reports on this work concerned the first year of life. Analysis of the video data at 3 months, 6 months and 9 months of age, confirmed that deaf mothers behaved differently to hearing mothers. Initially the study (at 3 months) discovered less signing by deaf mothers, and more vocalisations than expected (even with deaf infants); although signing increased at each point to 9 months. The data suggested

> "... deaf mothers are using less 'complex' and shorter utterances ... However, we must be careful here since the deaf mothers engage in a whole range of movement behaviours which subjectively look markedly different to hearing mothers."
>
> (Kyle, Woll & Ackerman, 1989, p. 37)

and also

> "… deaf mothers question less and report less but name considerably more and use no-sense[2] utterances more"   (p. 40)

and finally,

> "… We feel we should not try to avoid saying that deaf mothers use different strategies in an attempt to argue the case for their competence. Deaf mothers using sign do not have to follow the rules of hearing mothers in order to establish language competence in their children."   (p. 41–2)

Examining the data from the second year of life, it became clear that the interaction pattern of deaf and hearing mothers was different.

> "As the child's interest in the world around increases, the mother's control of infant's eye gaze becomes more difficult. For a hearing mother and child, the problem is less, because she can talk during object play. The deaf mother is faced with the task of gaining attention to give information and she needs to engage her child's attention before beginning to sign. We might predict that the deaf mother would engage in more overt attempts to break eye gaze to obtain the child's attention. … Deaf mothers achieve this training of attention by constantly placing themselves in a location to interrupt the child's line of gaze. Deaf mothers appear to view early interaction as a means of focussing the child's gaze and provide training in attention games. While this results in an apparently small amount of interaction and repetitive utterances when compared with hearing mothers, the result is the successful development of language at a comparable rate … to that of hearing children with hearing parents.   (p. 54)

These insights were novel and led directly to an intervention programme of training (Sutherland, 1983), where deaf parents visited homes of deaf children (with hearing parents) on a weekly basis to work on these significant aspects of adult–child interaction (applicable whether or not the child was going to be a sign user).

In a lexical analysis paper, more technical questions were addressed in relation to the development of signs in the second year of life.

> "The question becomes simpler: are we dealing with a proliferation of object signs or a series of symbolic object gestures? Are these simply analogous to the problems in determining words? … ["It is only during the second half of the second year … that discrete concepts are differentiated from the whole … (Nelson and Lucariello, 1985, p. 80) …] Such a change (from pre-lexical to lexical (denotational)) would allow us to incorporate both signs and meaningful symbolic gestures (and words)

---

2. Utterances which seemed ungrammatical or had no obvious meaning – later on considered to be in the "baby-sign" register.

into our data without being concerned about their ultimate status. In addition, it would explain the increase in solicit behaviour in the mothers in the second half of the first year: the game of naming is becoming more interesting for the child and the mother has less need to model." (Ackerman et al., 1990, p. 342)

The conclusion was becoming clear that deaf infants and children progressed to language mastery in BSL at a comparable rate to hearing children in speech, but as a result of different strategies by deaf caregivers. The responsibility to explain such strategies to hearing parent of deaf children was taken on by Ackerman and Sutherland through practical interaction with families. The insights gained by this process led to the setting up of the Deaf Children at Home project (for hearing parents) (Sutherland, 1983) and subsequently to the founding of a family centre for deaf children, whose development is described in the Stepping Stones report (Kyle et al., 2010).

As a partial aside to this work but arising directly from it, it is worth mentioning the less well-known paper in 1990, which set out the first steps in measuring deaf children's development of BSL. Kirk, Kyle, Ackerman and Woll (1990) set out a study of 80 children in four signing schools in the age range from 4 to 11 years and proposed a set of measures based on traditional receptive and productive vocabulary tests. Seven measures were introduced: baseline interview in BSL, order comprehension & production, classifier use, sign decomposition (rhyming), picture description, receptive vocabulary and expressive vocabulary. The paper described the challenges of adapting spoken language measures and trying to determine measurement which could be applied which would in future not require complete fluency in BSL in the adults administering the measures. Results were later reported separately and did not discover age effects, that is to say, older deaf children were not necessarily more advanced in BSL than younger children. The reasons for this the varying extent of exposure to sign language in deaf children from hearing families (and especially, the impossible task of determining how much signing was used at home). There was also the complication that while deaf assistants were present in the schools in the study, there was no way to determine how much interaction there was with the adult role model for individual deaf children. Since children were mostly day pupils, the extent of interaction among pupils was also variable. The notion of producing a "normed" test based on chronological age was abandoned at that time.

The final summary of this part of the initial work on acquisition came with the "Finding Out" report to the research council in 2004. The report focused on the emergence of questions in the recordings of the deaf children who had been followed since a few months old. The following is the summary of the primary analysis of the data:

The results indicate that BSL questions do not seem to develop earlier than spoken English questions as was predicted and they do not follow the pattern of adult questions. There appears to be no interrogative function in early question interaction and questions are signalled more as turn-taking. The terminal hold of sign utterances is taken to be a question marker in both adult and child signing.

An extension of this work with the same children several years later confirmed the presence of adult signed question forms but did not provide a simple model of their acquisition. This was seen even more strikingly in elicitation tasks with Deaf schoolchildren from hearing families.

The conclusion which we can now make is that the syntactic and pragmatic aspects of question formation are treated differently in signed questions and that the pattern of acquisition is not as neatly laid out as had been anticipated. Facial expressions associated with questions are separate from the syntax of questions. It appears that it is not the use of a wh-feature which determines whether or not a given non-manual marker is used. What is crucial is the pragmatic condition of a question.

These insights were carried over into Bencie Woll's work from 2005 onwards at DCAL, which is further described in other chapters in this volume.

Impact

It should be clear that the work that Bencie Woll has carried out in this field has been of great significance. Starting in 1978, with almost no research work on BSL and with deaf people seen as a backward, isolated and handicapped group, the progress has been enormous. The account above has been selective dealing with the early years and trying to give an indication of how it all started. It is not complete: for example, it does not cover work on the teaching of sign language, on research on interpreter training nor on television, but it has tried to draw on less well-known papers and presentations of which those working in Deaf Studies may be less aware.

The evidence base in the rest of this book has expanded far beyond these early projects and some of Bencie's insights can be seen to have been modified and enhanced over time. Bencie Woll created a firm foundation upon which she and other researchers were able to build. Sign Language Studies was able to emerge from the wilderness of the 1970s and become a significant addition into the fields of language development and linguistics.

References

Ackerman, J., Kyle J. G., Woll, B., & Ezra, M. (1990). Lexical acquisition in sign and speech. In C. Lucas (Ed.), *Sign language research: Theoretical issues*. Washington, DC: Gallaudet University Press.

Brennan, M. (1976). Can deaf children acquire language? *Supplement to the British Deaf News*. Carlisle: BDA.

Conrad, R. (1979). *The deaf school child*. London: Harper and Row.

Dale, D. M. C. (1974). *Language development in deaf and partially hearing children*. Springfield, IL: Charles C. Thomas.

Deuchar, M. (1978). *Diglossia and British Sign Language* (Unpublished PhD dissertation). Stanford University.

Evans, L. (1982). *Total communication: Structure and strategy*. Washington, DC: Gallaudet University Press.

Kirk, B., Kyle, J. G., Ackerman, J., & Woll, B. (1990). Measuring British Sign Language development in deaf children. In J. Kyle (Ed.), *Deafness and sign language into the 1990s*. Bristol: Deaf Studies Trust.

Kyle, J. G., Williamson, T., Dawson, N., Willoughby, A., Canavan, M., Cheskin, A., & Palmer, N. (2010). *Stepping stones: Family responses to services provided to their deaf children*. Bristol: Family Centre and Deaf Studies Trust. <http://www.deafstudiestrust.org/downloads.php>

Kyle, J. G., & Woll, B. (1983). *Language in sign: An international perspective on sign language*. London: Croom Helm.

Kyle, J. G., & Woll, B. (2004). *Finding out: Developing questions in BSL, final report to ESRC, for ESRC*. Bristol: Centre for Deaf Studies.

Kyle, J. G., Woll, B., & Ackerman, J. (1989). *From gesture to sign and speech: Final report to ESRC*. Bristol: School of Education.

Kyle, J. G., Woll, B., & Ackerman, J. (1989). Gesture to sign and speech, final report to ESRC, Project No: C00-23-2327. Bristol: School of Education Research Unit.

Lewis, M. M. (1968). *The education of deaf children: The possible place of fingerspelling and signing*. London: HMSO.

Nelson, K., and Lucariello, J. (1985). The development of meaning in first word speech, pp 59–86, In M. D. Barrett (Ed.), *Children's Single Word Speech*. London: Wiley.

Stokoe, W. C. (1960). *Sign language structure: An outline of the visual communication system of the American deaf* (Studies in Linguistics Occasional Paper 8). Buffalo, NY: University of Buffalo.

Sutherland, H. (1983). *Deaf children at home*. Bristol: Centre for Deaf Studies. <http://www.deafstudiestrust.org/downloads.php>

Tylor, E. B. (1874). *Researches into the early history of mankind*. London: Murray.

Wells, G. (1981). *Learning through interaction*. Cambridge: Cambridge University Press.

Woll, B., Kyle, J. G., & Deuchar, M. (1981). *Perspectives on British Sign Language and deafness*. London: Croom Helm.

Woll, B., & Lawson, L. (1980). British Sign Language. Paper presented at the 1st International Symposium on Minority Languages, Glasgow: September 1980. In E. Haugen, J. D. McClure, & B. S. Thomson (Eds.), *Minority languages today*. Edinburgh: EUP.

CHAPTER 1

Deafness, cognition and language
Developmental perspectives

Gary Morgan

This opening chapter sets the scene for the volume by describing in the first
section what researchers mean by a native user of a signed language, and what
differences exist between the deaf child who has deaf parents and those in the
vast majority of cases from hearing families. This experience of late or reduced
exposure to accessible language can have far reaching consequences and in this
introduction chapter the areas of early interaction and later cognitive development are highlighted. The second half of the chapter describes the contents
of the book by summarizing the key findings from each chapter. The chapter
concludes with some future research questions for language development
research that follow on from this volume.

Aims of this book

Deafness impacts on children in many ways and the most obvious is in the acquisition of language. There has been much written over the past decades and even
centuries about how being born deaf influences a child's natural development of
language (Lane, 1984). This is surprising in one way, as the incidence rate of congenital deafness is very low in the population (1–2 per 1000). At the same time, it
is not surprising why so much attention has been devoted to this group. Deafness
and language development is very interesting because in the majority of cases
language delay ensues not because of general cognitive development difficulties
but because of the child's environment. As Hans Furth pointed out in 1966, the
majority of deaf children have the same non-verbal IQ and intellectual potential as
hearing children but this potential is very rarely realised.

The second reason why deafness is so popular a topic in our field of language
development is because it also sets up interesting questions concerning what impact
language development delay has on linked cognitive skills (e.g. Theory of Mind).
The current volume thus concerns what we know about how deafness affects both

https://doi.org/10.1075/tilar.25.01mor

cognitive and language development. The volume also describes and marks the contribution of Bencie Woll to our field. It is special for any researcher to have such a big impact in a single area of study such as deafness and development. It is rarer still to see how a researcher such as Bencie Woll has influenced several linked fields – sign language linguistics, neuroscience, psycholinguistics and clinical and educational language research – to such an extent. While we touch on some of these linked topics, the main focus is on developmental issues in deafness.

Changes in how deaf children are learning language

It is interesting to note that Bencie Woll began work as a researcher in the field of language development on the Gordon Wells (1986) project 'Meaning Makers' in Bristol, UK (see Jim Kyle's description of this in the foreword). She later applied much of that early work to the first studies of BSL development. In several early projects, Woll and colleagues at Bristol attempted to describe how early interaction might be influenced by the situation where one or both of the child and adult is deaf and uses a signed language. This early work stimulated a line of research on parent-child interaction described in Chapters 2 and 3. Much later, in 2002, Bencie and I were asked to edit the second volume in the TiLAR series titled *Directions in Signed Language Acquisition* (Morgan & Woll, 2002). That volume grew in part, out of the early work in Bristol and the set of chapters it contained reflected how Bencie Woll's work on language acquisition chimed with an international group of researchers. That volume concentrated mostly on describing native sign language acquisition. Perhaps at this point in the current volume it would be good to define what is meant by a native signer as it will be appearing in several other chapters as well.

Who are native signers?

In spoken language development the vast majority of children become native speakers of at least one language (and in many cases more than one) by the simple fact that they have an extended period of time exposed to fluent language models – the native speakers of their community. The main requirement for becoming a native speaker is that the child is exposed to early and consistent input in that language (i.e. typically the child acquires the language of the adults around them from birth). While this is for the most part unproblematic for hearing children acquiring spoken language (see Lillo-Martin, Smith, & Tsimpli, this volume), it is a very complicated situation when the child is born deaf. This is because the vast majority of deaf children are born to parents who are fluent speakers of a spoken language (and not a signed language). Early interaction and communication is reported in many studies to be difficult when for the first few years deaf children find spoken language effortful to learn (see Harris & Clibbens, this volume). This difficulty has been reducing with the advent of neo-natal screening for deafness and technological interventions such as early Cochlear Implants (CI), but there is still wide variability in the ultimate attainment of spoken language skills of deaf children. This situation is coupled with exposure to signed language typically being very late in the case of deaf children of hearing parents, often being learned only as a fall-back option at school or not at all during childhood (and thus beyond the typical 'sensitive' period for language development).

Describing why there are differences between being a native or non-native speaker has several controversial theoretical implications. Two very important ones being: (1) Is language under the influence of a biological critical period? (2) How does the quality and quantity of input influence the course of development? Only a small percentage of deaf children (5–10%) are born to parents who are fluent speakers of a signed language. This means that the children typically experience early exposure to a signed language, and thus develop language following well-attested stages of development and are termed native signers. The vast majority of research on sign language and sign language development has been carried out with native signers, despite these children being the atypical case.

The focus by researchers on children who have been exposed to a natural signed language by their deaf parents facilitated signed language acquisition as a field within language development studies. Over the years, work in this area has been growing, and reached a significant high point following the inclusion of a chapter (Newport & Meier, 1985) on American Sign Language (ASL) in Dan Slobin's volumes on cross-linguistic acquisition. Another major catalyst for the study of native signers was Ursula Bellugi, a student of Roger Brown, who subsequently began conducting systematic psycholinguistic studies of ASL, including those of language acquisition, in the research programme at the Salk Institute. There was always an impetus in Newport, Meier and Bellugi's early research projects to treat native signers as a typical example of language development.

At the same time, many deaf children do not become any type of signer (not native or non-native) because they are exposed to uniquely spoken languages. These children in the literature have typically been referred to as 'oral' deaf children. Several chapters in this book document the effects on development of different exposure to signing or oral languages.

Oral versus signed language exposure

Research on language development in deaf children covers two main areas of focus. One has concentrated on investigating the acquisition of signed languages in both native signers (deaf children of deaf parents) as well as the deaf children of hearing parents who were learning a signed language. In the past, deaf children with hearing parents typically did not learn a signed language from birth, but rather learned signed language at different ages in childhood and even in adolescence through attending the large number of schools for the deaf. As Tang and colleagues (this volume) document, the majority of deaf schools in the early days had an exclusively oral approach. From the 1970s onwards, education standards were generally low and did not seem to be improving; thus the idea of introducing signed language into school became more popular. For example, the realisation that reading attainment was very poor despite an exclusive focus on oral language proficiency in the school meant other options had to be investigated (Conrad, 1979). From the 1980s onwards there was a growth in programmes available for parents to learn sign in an attempt to foster better home communication. However, more recently (over the past 15 years) the landscape has begun to change in that the number of special schools for the deaf has decreased dramatically – not because of a reduction in the number of deaf children, but as a preference for mainstreaming children. Similarly, resources made available for parents or professionals to learn sign to communicate with deaf children has reduced. At the same time the number of deaf children who were taking more easily to spoken languages has increased because of early interventions made possible through neonatal screening for deafness and better quality digital hearing aids and early CIs.

The other area of focus of research into childhood deafness has been the acquisition of spoken languages (in 'oral' deaf children), with an emphasis on documenting differences in acquisition of spoken language between deaf children and their hearing peers (Marschark & Spencer, 2006). In this context, deaf children are exposed to the spoken language of their parents but their deafness means that their access to this input is severely limited. Thus, these children typically experience incomplete development of their native language. In the past, differences between deaf and hearing children's spoken language skills were very large. In recent years – again because of neonatal screening, better interventions and improved access to sound by CIs / hearing aids – these differences have narrowed, but not for all children.

While changes in neo-natal screening, school setting and CIs are changing the lives of young deaf children, we do not know what the future impact will be on language and cognitive development. Currently, researchers are witnessing a very big change in the language used by deaf children. Deaf children of deaf parents continue to acquire signed languages, and a number of hearing parents expose their deaf children at different points in their development to a signed language. However, both groups are also increasingly being exposed to spoken language either solely, or else before, after, or at the same time as being exposed to signed language. While outcomes for acquiring spoken language are improving across the board, there is still a lot of variability unaccounted for.

These diverse contexts have led to several interesting research questions in language development research, including:

1. How does deafness impact on the early foundations of language development?
2. How much early language exposure is enough to become a native speaker or signer?
3. What are the long-term outcomes of late language exposure?

What does deafness/modality mean for related cognitive skills and brain plasticity?

While the development of language in deaf children has been studied for several decades, a growing parallel field has looked at how deafness might affect children's cognitive skills. Note that many cognitive differences between deaf and hearing children might be the result of co-morbidity between the causes of the deafness and the causes of delays in memory, attention, and other cognitive skills. This makes studying relationships between language and cognition difficult. The issue of how language and cognition can be separated is a thorny one because many aspects of cognition and language are intertwined in processing, development and attainment on cognitive assessments (see Cardin & colleagues, this volume).

Despite this caveat, a hallmark of studies that look at deaf children's cognition is that the participants generally have normal development of non-verbal abilities. Michael Siegal and Candida Peterson made the interesting point that deaf children of hearing parents most often pass false photo tests at the same age as typically-developing hearing peers, indicating that they have appropriate symbolic representation skills. However, these same children are significantly delayed in passing the false belief test, and in general find it difficult to represent false beliefs (Peterson & Siegal, 1998). So why does late language development affect higher aspects of cognitive development? It might be that it is only in the interface between later cognitive development (e.g., problem solving) where reduced language skills impacts cognition. There are two ways in which growing up deaf in a surrounding hearing family might impact on cognition: (1) through delayed exposure to language, and (2) through a reduced exposure to information around the deaf child from hearing parents (access to world knowledge). This second aspect was first descried, by Furth (1966) as a 'narrowing' of cognitive experience.

Note that the inclusion of a group of native signers in many studies allows us to discount the audiological effects of deafness on cognition and focus more on the subsequent effects deafness has for access to natural language development and access to wider information. When a language delay has been avoided by the child acquiring a native command of a signed language, a switch to a different modality appears to not disrupt the typical milestones of higher-level cognitive development. Two areas that have received much research are between native and non-native signers development of Theory of Mind (ToM, e.g. Woolfe, Want & Siegal, 2002) and Executive Functions (EF, e.g. Hall, Eigsti, Bortfeld, & Lillo-Martin, 2018). In both these areas, we can see how studying deafness tells us a great deal about the importance of early communication and language in higher-level cognitive development.

In several ToM studies access to conversation about mental states has been suggested to facilitate the child's speed in attaining the typical milestones of social cognition (de Rosnay et al., 2014). In a linked area – pragmatics – we see that even with dramatic improvements in spoken language skills, some young deaf children find the social pragmatic skills needed for understanding interactions very difficult (highlighted in the work of Peterson & Siegal, 1998). Thus in some aspects of social-pragmatic development, deaf children continue to experience difficulties despite advances in language development.

In another area of higher cognitive skills – (Executive Functions) – deafness seems to play a very important role (see Morgan, Jones, & Botting, this volume). Exactly why deaf children have poorer EFs than normally-hearing children is debated in the literature. One possibility is that the reduced access to sound impedes EF development – known as the Auditory Scaffolding Hypothesis (e.g., Pisoni, Conway, Kronenberger, Henning, & Anaya, 2010). This proposes that processing of sequential signals of sound and spoken language sets up and develops EFs. Some have pointed out that this account might not be applicable to all deaf children: deaf native signers appear to have age-appropriate development of EF, suggesting that it might not be only a sound-based language signal which can scaffold cognitive control (Hall et al., 2018). However, deaf children with hearing parents who are acquiring spoken language or a mixture of signs and speech do seem to have delayed EF development. A second possibility to explain poorer EFs in deaf children might be an early reduction in emotional-cognitive regulation provided by scaffolded interactions, or the lack of sufficient linguistic inner speech necessary to do EF tasks on-line.

While there is undoubtedly a positive impact of early sign (language) exposure from deaf parents, there remains a gap in our understanding of whether hearing parents are able to achieve a sufficient level of early communication and language skills in order to facilitate the same levels of development. The data to date suggest this is in general a difficult challenge, but we are still trying to understand 'how much is enough' exposure and for how long this early sign exposure needs to be present. This is important because both language and cognitive development are the foundation stones of children's future academic achievement. The fact that the majority of deaf children continue to have a varied amount of language and cognitive delays means that their school learning will be compromised. Many researchers have argued that the large achievement gap between deaf and hearing children is unacceptable. However, without the necessary optimal language and cognitive tools with which to learn, deaf children will continue to have suboptimal achievement.

Deaf children's changing experience of education

Deafness has been studied for many years as a test case in developmental psychology for evaluating what intrinsic abilities and constraints children possess. However, over recent years researchers have turned their attention to how research can improve what we know about how deaf children learn, with the ultimate aim of improving their academic attainment (Marschark & Hauser, 2011). This is linked with the need to understand how the environment (especially the school experience) can shape development. There has always been a conundrum in deaf education in that while deaf children educated in deaf schools (for the most part in isolation from hearing communities) meant that signed language could be acquired through informal contact with deaf peers, but academic achievements were not generally high. The conundrum is: what is the purpose of school, social stimulation or academic achievement? In the UK, *The Report of the Committee of Enquiry into the Education of Handicapped Children and Young People in the UK*, chaired by Mary Warnock and published in 1978, stimulated a gradual reduction in deaf-only schools and a move towards the integration of deaf children in wider education (mainstreaming). The argument is that deaf children learn more when they are surrounded by hearing children but an increased focus on mainstreaming can lead to increased possible social exclusion. However, the evidence for better educational attainment based on a deaf school or mainstreaming model is perplexingly missing (Knoors & Marschark, 2012).

At the same time, it is very difficult to arrive at an answer as to what type of school is optimal for a deaf child. In fact, the answer could possibly be 'the one that currently suits the child best'. This means that there might need to be several options available to parents and their children and that the child might need to transition between them at different points in development. However, for the study of deafness, cognition and language development, we know very little about how these educational influences will facilitate or hinder deaf children's learning. As with wider comparisons of different types of speech and language therapy, studies in education and deafness are hampered by a general reluctance from researchers to both evaluate interventions in existence and/or carry out intervention studies themselves. Finding out what works (or does not work well) is very difficult and, at times, can produce uncomfortable findings.

What is in the book?

With this context laid out, we now turn to the contents of the current volume. As described in the Foreword by Jim Kyle, there has been a steadily growing realisation in our field that the early foundations of parent–child interaction will sow the seeds for a set of future developments. For example, in research on hearing infants it is suggested that children who are stimulated to be more active in learning about their environment and whose parents positively scaffolding their actions with contingent language show the most EF benefits (e.g., Devine, Bignardi, & Hughes, 2016). Thus, understanding the dynamics of early communication in deaf and hearing children is essential. Chapter 2 by Margaret Harris and John Clibbens considers the similarities and differences between visual and auditory communication, focusing on early child–caregiver communication, and showing how understanding of this phenomenon has unfolded over several decades of research. In the first part of the chapter they identify the key characteristics of effective infant–caregiver communication, focusing particularly on the development of joint attention, and outlining what is required for infants to perceive, interpret, and respond to early linguistic and nonverbal communication. They also review evidence of interventions to provide direct support for infant–caretaker interactions to see whether appropriate advice and guidance can improve the quality of interactions with young deaf children.

In Chapter 3, Anne Baker and Beppie van den Bogaerde analyse the nuances of early interaction and turn-taking patterns in deaf children with deaf parents. Basing their analysis on adult turn-taking systems, they outline how both overlap occurring in conversations and modality-specific attention-getting strategies play a role in gaining and holding a turn. The data come from three native signers: mother–child dyads (2 to 6 years) and one mother–child triad (twins, 5 years old) in spontaneous interaction in Sign Language of the Netherlands. The authors describe the patterns and regularities in how interaction unfolds and how this is acquired over time. They describe how adult attention-getting strategies change from being mainly implicit to increasingly explicit strategies and discuss reasons for this change. The children are apparently learning to use the 'collaborative floor', which they will need in adult–adult signed conversation.

Chapter 4 by Rosalind Herman, Nicola Grove, Tobias Haug, Wolfgang Mann and Philip Prinz focuses on the assessment of signed language. In the wider field of language acquisition, the main impetus has been to understand *how* the child learns language and also to develop tools for the assessment of the group of hearing children with language developmental delays. In the study of deaf children's signed language development those endeavors have also gone hand-in-hand. Much research has described the typical case of native sign development, but then used this information to inform how an assessment tool could be constructed to measure development in a diverse set of children (mostly late learners). Despite the large number of assessments available to measure spoken language acquisition, until relatively recently no assessments were available that could be used to evaluate deaf children's sign language acquisition. Development of signed language assessments presents unique methodological challenges. The chapter focuses on (i) the issues involved in designing signed language assessments, including the design of web-based assessments, and (ii) the use of static and dynamic signed language assessments with diverse groups of signed language users, ranging from deaf children to typically-developing hearing adults learning signed language as an L2 and hearing adults with intellectual disabilities who use sign to communicate.

In Chapter 5, Chloë Marshall, Katherine Rowley, Joanna Atkinson, Tanya Denmark, Joanna Hoskins & Jechil Sieratzki describe how the early work of Bencie Woll has focused on what the study of signed language and atypical signers who have neurological differences teaches us about language and cognition more generally. At the same time as the general field of language development was describing typical language development, a growing group of researchers was documenting why some hearing children exposed to spoken language from birth were experiencing severe difficulties in learning to communicate. The goals were to understand how Specific Language Impairment (SLI), now referred to as Developmental Language Disorder (DLD), could help explain typical development as well as understand what was disrupted in atypical language development. The same motivations were present in the growing field of atypical signed language development. The chapter reviews the literature showing that studies of atypical users of language allow us to gain insights into typical development more generally. The authors provide an overview of developmental research on individuals and small-groups with Specific Language Impairment, Autistic Spectrum Disorder including a case of a linguistic savant, William's Syndrome, Down syndrome, Landau-Kleffner Syndrome, Tourette's syndrome and Stuttering. The chapter ends by considering the role for deaf practitioners and fluent signing therapists in the development of signed language therapy for children who are atypical signers.

Returning to the issue of native signers, Chapter 6 by Diane Lillo-Martin, Neil Smith, and Ianthi Tsimpli describes age of acquisition effects in signed language development. The authors explore in detail how language acquisition by deaf children can be complicated, compared to typical monolingual development of spoken languages. Late first-language acquisition of a signed language reveals that age-of-acquisition effects (i.e., the age at which an individual is exposed to a language) must be taken into consideration as linguistic theories of acquisition are refined. Age of acquisition effects in spoken languages differ between vocabulary and grammar; whereas there appears to be no sensitive period for acquiring a vocabulary, the acquisition of grammar appears time sensitive and thus native-like attainment is difficult for individuals who have comparatively late exposure (Hartshorne, Tenenbaum & Pinker, 2018). In signed language development, parallel differentiations can be expected between the acquisition of syntax as opposed to the acquisition of the sign lexicon. In addition, few deaf children who acquire a signed language are purely monolingual; instead, they are generally bilingual (to different extents) in a signed language and a spoken language (bimodal bilingualism). When spoken language is accessed through a cochlear implant, age of acquisition effects can again be seen, and the presence or absence of signed language is an important factor. Finally, the development of a signed language as a second language in unique contexts such as that of Christopher, a polyglot savant, can reveal more about the nature of language development and the theories of language structure that must be posited to account for the full range of circumstances under which signed languages may be acquired.

Turning from language development, the next chapter integrates what we understand about how deaf children's signed and spoken language development relates to cognitive domains. In Chapter 7, Gary Morgan, Anna Jones and Nicola Botting describe why language development is crucial for deaf children's cognitive development, with particular focus on the role of language for Theory of Mind development and Executive Functions. This chapter explores the notion of what it means for a deaf child to become a communicative partner with a hearing parent, and how children learn signed languages when their parents are typically hearing. These issues are couched in terms of how early interaction might shape language development, and how cognitive skills support and are linked to communicative experience.

The following chapter extends this work on cognitive development to describe in wider detail a range of psycholinguistic processes linked to deafness and the comprehension and production of signing. Matthew Dye and Robin Thompson outline how the field of language processing seeks to understand the psychological processes that underpin the production and comprehension of language. The current understanding of how these processes work is tied predominantly to spoken languages; the authors show how psycholinguistic research of signed languages can inform us about processes specific to the visual-manual modality and what this means for language acquisition by deaf children. The chapter details the latest research on sign language processing using eye-tracking technology and relates this to the task of acquiring a signed language. The authors raise the issue of how early in the development of visual cognition a child needs to 'see' a signed language in order to make the important link between language and attention.

Inherent in this work is the idea that the cognitive and brain systems used during language acquisition have to adapt to the change in signal from the default of sound to the visual modality. This is the topic of Chapter 9 on brain plasticity and language development by Velia Cardin, Ruth Campbell, Mairéad MacSweeney, Emil Holmer, Jerker Rönnberg and Mary Rudner. The authors begin by outlining the importance of 'sensitive periods' and the impact of deafness in early life on the reorganisation dictated by vision and somato-sensation. Deaf individuals will develop visual strategies for language, and in many cases language acquisition will be delayed. This means that there is also a difference in the early language experience of deaf and hearing individuals. The chapter reviews the neural reorganisation that occurs as a consequence of deafness per se, and relates that to differences in language use and acquisition.

Finally, in Chapter 10 Gladys Tang, Robert Adam and Karen Simpson focus on the current understanding of how signed language can be incorporated into the education of deaf children. The authors begin by describing the history of signed languages used in schools and then describe current practice, as well as outlining challenges to sign bilingual education. These include the reduction in children who are exposed to signed language in schools, as well as the language contact situation (spoken and signed languages mixed). As the default has become inclusive education for deaf children, interaction in the classroom and daily communication between hearing and deaf children may lead to a variety of types of signings. The authors argue for increased research into the impact of this mixture of signing inputs on acquisition, processing and ultimately educational attainment.

The book closes with an Afterword by Ruth Campbell, which describes how the past study of deaf children focused on a readership within an educational or clinical setting, but makes the important point that this field has now become much wider in its remit. At the same time, the majority of research in the past on language development and processing was based on hearing people as participants. Campbell describes how research led by Bencie Woll and others has transformed the small field of deafness into what it constitutes today – an important link to several mainstream fields, especially language acquisition. The next stages of research into deafness, cognition and language are set to open up even more interesting but complex questions. Campbell points to a set of outstanding issues including the following: Which neural circuits are used to process signed and spoken language, and how is this influenced by the social environment in which the child develops? How does late and impoverished language acquisition impact on cognitive, communicative and linguistic performance? Finally, what will be the consequences of the current changes in how the medical field treats deafness and the educational field educates deaf children?

At the outset of this chapter, we pointed out that few fields are influenced by a single person as much as ours has been. Bencie Woll would be the first to acknowledge that her work has been the outcome of fruitful collaborations with many colleagues. However, as the chapters in this volume attest, Bencie has been able to bring together a deep theoretical interest in the brain and development with an honest wish to influence practice in the classroom, clinic and family. Her work stands out as a model of how deaf and hearing people can collaborate together successfully. She has developed a strong field that spreads across Europe and other parts of the world, as well as incorporates insights from several disciplines. In all of this, Bencie never lost sight of the need to anticipate future changes to our field. And thus, this volume is both dedicated to her ideas and is a testament to the indelible mark she has made on the rapidly evolving field of deaf children's language and cognitive development.

References

Conrad, R. (1979). *The deaf school child*. London: Harper & Row.

De Rosnay, M., Fink, E., Begeer, S., Slaughter, V., & Peterson, C. (2014). Talking theory of mind talk: Young school-aged children's everyday conversation and understanding of mind and emotion. *Journal of Child Language* 41, 1179–1193.
https://doi.org/10.1017/S0305000913000433

Devine, R. T., Bignardi, G., & Hughes, C. (2016). Executive function mediates the relations between parental behaviors and children's early academic ability. *Frontiers in Psychology* 7, 1902. https://doi.org/10.3389/fpsyg.2016.01902

Furth, H. G. (1966). *Thinking without language. Psychological implications of deafness*. New York, NY: The Free Press.

Hall, M. L., Eigsti, I.-M., Bortfeld, H., & Lillo-Martin, D. (2018). Executive function in deaf children: Auditory access and language access. *Journal of Speech, Language, and Hearing Research*. https://doi.org/10.1044/2018_JSLHR-L-17-0281

Hartshorne, J. K., Tenenbaum, J. B., & Pinker, S. (2018). A critical period for second language acquisition: Evidence from 2/3 million English speakers. *Cognition* 177, 263–277.
https://doi.org/10.1016/j.cognition.2018.04.007

Knoors, H. & Marschark, M. (2012). Language planning for the 21st Century: Revisiting bilingual language policy for deaf children. *The Journal of Deaf Studies and Deaf Education* 17, 291–305. https://doi.org/10.1093/deafed/ens018

Lane, H. (1984). *When the mind hears: A history of the deaf.* New York, NY: Random House.

Marschark, M., & Spencer, P. E. (2006). Spoken language development of deaf and hard-of-hearing children: Historical and theoretical perspectives. In P. E. Spencer & M. Marschark (Eds.), *Perspectives on deafness. Advances in the spoken language development of deaf and hard-of-hearing children* (pp. 3–21). Oxford: Oxford University Press.

Marschark, M., & Hauser, P. (2011). *How deaf children learn: What parents and teachers need to know.* Oxford: Oxford University Press.

Morgan, G., & Woll, B. (Eds.). (2002). *Directions in sign language acquisition.* Amsterdam: John Benjamins. https://doi.org/10.1075/tilar.2

Newport, E. L., & Meier, R. P. (1985). The acquisition of American Sign Language. In D. I. Slobin (Ed.), *The cross-linguistic study of language acquisition* (Vol. 1, pp. 881–938). Hillsdale, NJ: Lawrence Erlbaum Associates.

Peterson, C., & Siegal, M. (1998). Changing focus on the representational mind: Concepts of false photos, false drawings and false beliefs in deaf, autistic and normal children. *British Journal of Developmental Psychology* 16, 301–320.
https://doi.org/10.1111/j.2044-835X.1998.tb00754.x

Pisoni, D. B., Conway, C. M., Kronenberger, W. G., Henning, S., & Anaya, E. (2010). Executive function, cognitive control, and sequence learning in deaf children with cochlear implants. In M. Marschark & P. E. Spencer (Eds.), *Oxford handbook of deaf studies, language, and education* (Vol. 2). New York, NY: Oxford University Press.
https://doi.org/10.1093/oxfordhb/9780195390032.013.0029

Slobin, D. I. (Ed.). (1985). *The crosslinguistic study of language acquisition* Vol. 1. The data; Vol. 2. Theoretical issues (pp. 881–938). Hillsdale, NJ: Lawrence Erlbaum Associates.

Warnock Report. (1978). *Special educational needs.* London: HMSO.

Wells, G. (1986). *The meaning makers: Learning to talk and talking to learn.* Clevedon: Multilingual Matters.

Woolfe, T., Want, S., & Siegal, M. (2002). Signposts to development: Theory of mind in deaf children. *Child Development* 73, 768–778. https://doi.org/10.1111/1467-8624.00437

Early communication in deaf and hearing children

Margaret Harris and John Clibbens

This chapter considers the similarities and differences between visual and auditory communication, focusing on early communication between infants and young children and their caretakers and showing how understanding of this phenomenon has unfolded over several decades of research. We identify key characteristics of effective infant–caretaker communication, focusing particularly on the development of joint attention. We explain how the dynamics of early communication can be affected by the hearing status of the infant and the caretaker and we review evidence from interventions that provide direct support for infant–caretaker interactions. Finally, we compare outcomes for the current cohort of deaf infants with those born before recent innovations in diagnosis and hearing aid technology.

We first began researching early interaction between deaf mothers and their deaf infants in the early 1980s. At the time there was very little published research on the topic but we discovered that Bencie Woll and Jim Kyle, who were then working at the Centre for Deaf Studies at the University of Bristol, had begun work on this very topic. We contacted Bencie and she invited us to visit them and see the Centre. We learned an enormous amount from our initial and subsequent conversations with Bencie, especially about the importance of involving native signers in our research. Thanks to Bencie's considerable networking skills, we also found out about other researchers who were starting to think about deaf mother–infant interaction. In the years that followed we often met Bencie to talk about research and share ideas. She was always enthusiastic about the latest research findings and the picture that was slowly emerging of the way that deaf mothers interacted with their infants and how this impacted on the early stages of sign language development. Bencie also became interested in the development of a standardised measure of early British Sign Language (BSL) vocabulary and she realised this objective as one of the authors of the first BSL adaptation of the Communicative Development Inventories (CDI) (Woolfe, Herman, Roy, & Woll, 2010).

https://doi.org/10.1075/tilar.25.02har

In this chapter we reflect on major research findings from the last three decades. We consider the similarities and differences between visual and auditory communication, focusing on early communication between infants and young children (up to the age of 3 years) and their caretakers, and discuss how understanding of this phenomenon has unfolded over many years of research. In the first part of the chapter we identify the key characteristics of effective infant–caretaker communication, focusing particularly on the development of joint attention, and we show what is required for infants to perceive, interpret and respond to early linguistic and nonverbal communication. We explain how the dynamics of early communication can be affected by the hearing status of the infant and the caretaker and we compare the communication patterns of deaf and hearing caretakers with deaf and hearing infants. In the second part of the chapter we consider the impact of universal newborn hearing screening and the availability of cochlear implants and digital hearing aids on early communication. We compare outcomes for the current cohort of deaf infants with those born before the advent of these technological innovations and we consider how early infant–caretaker communication can change following cochlear implantation. Finally, we review evidence of interventions to provide direct support for infant–caretaker interactions to see whether appropriate advice and guidance can improve the quality of interactions with young deaf children.

Joint attention and early language

The earliest communication between infants and their caretakers involves a great deal of mutual gaze. This early interaction is often described as dyadic (i.e., two-way) and, over time, it becomes increasingly complex as infants and their caretakers develop oft-repeated social routines that involve everyday activities such as feeding and bath time, or simple games such as 'peekaboo'. These social routines, which begin in the first months of life, are repeated many times over the course of a day and this repetition allows the infant to become an increasingly active partner, gradually learning to anticipate the next step in the sequence. Routines of this kind can be observed in both deaf and hearing infants; and parents who sign are likely to incorporate signs and gestures into the routines just as parents who use spoken language will incorporate words and gestures (Spencer & Harris, 2006).

Young children's growing familiarity with games and routines plays an important part in the learning of early language, (Bruner, 1975, 1983; Scaife & Bruner, 1975). According to Bruner, infants' developing knowledge of social routines allows them to build up insights into the meaning of the words that, alongside gestures and facial expressions, adults use as part of these familiar routines. Children's early understanding of words is often associated with specific dyadic routines but, somewhere between 6 and 9 months, there is an important development in patterns of social interaction that provides a new opportunity for language development. At this age, infants become increasingly interested in objects or events in the environment and interaction with caretakers becomes increasingly triadic (i.e., three-way), involving caretaker, child and the environment (Bakeman & Adamson, 1984). The development of triadic interaction affords an important opportunity for infant and caretaker to share joint attention with the external world.

Since the concept of triadic joint attention was first characterized by Bakeman and Adamson there has been considerable debate about exactly what it means for infant and caretaker to share attention. Is it merely necessary for both partners to attend to the same thing or is it also necessary that both partners *know together* that they are attending to the same thing (Tomasello, 1995)? The difference is between *parallel attention*, in which two individuals are looking at the same thing, and *joint attention*, in which both individuals know that the other is sharing attention. There are a number of indicators of this latter kind of joint attention in young children. These include looking up at an adult and then back to a shared object, pointing at an object and then looking to the adult and, a few months later, the use of language to refer to the common focus of attention. Recent research suggests that, whereas human infants engage in truly joint attention, chimpanzees and other apes do not (Carpenter & Call, 2013). Only human infants are capable of sharing attention and they will repeat an action until an adult acknowledges this. For example, if an adult responds to the pointing of a 12-month-old by speaking enthusiastically to the infant but ignoring the object, the infant will point again at the same object. However, if the adult responds by speaking enthusiastically and alternating gaze between the object and the infant, infants do not repeat the point (Liszkowski, Carpenter, Henning, Striano, & Tomasello, 2004).

The understanding and use of pointing provides one way in which infant and caretaker can know together that they are attending to the same object or event. Pointing provides a way for communicative partners to clearly establish a joint frame of reference (Butterworth, 2001) and, potentially, for infants to learn the meaning of the many labels that adults produce when their children point. Indeed, there is a correlation between the age at which infants first start to point and their emerging understanding that objects have names (Harris, Barlow-Brown, & Chasin, 1995). However, the use of pointing to a distant object presents particular difficulties for children who do not have access to spoken language because of their deafness. When they turn to look at the object being pointed at, they can no longer see their caretaker. For a child who can hear, this presents no difficulty but for a deaf child, who needs to be looking at the caretaker in order to see what is being signed or said (via speech reading), pointing can present a significant challenge for word learning.

Joint attention in deaf children

A wealth of studies has highlighted some notable differences in the dynamics of joint attention for deaf and hearing children that have implications for early language development. The early studies typically focused on deaf children who had little or no benefit from early amplification (Spencer & Harris, 2006). For these children, who have very restricted access to speech in the early years, effective communication cannot make use of the auditory channel and is predominantly visual. Thus, the opportunities for these children to learn language relies on both the object of joint attention and its verbal label being perceived through the visual modality, thereby creating a potential need for deaf children to divide attention between caretaker and object. Such divided attention is thought to be problematic for early word learning which relies on 'contingent naming', that is, the simultaneous availability of an object and its verbal label. If a child has to look away from the object of attention in order to see a signed label, this makes it less likely that the child will see the two as contingent because they cannot be observed at exactly the same time. Evidence from hearing children shows that the precise timing of object labelling by adults is of great importance for early word learning and early vocabulary development can be delayed if the child cannot hear an object label and, and the same time, see the relevant object (Harris, Jones, Brookes, & Grant, 1986).

Research into the signing strategies of mothers of young deaf children – and particularly mothers who are deaf themselves – suggested that many of the potential problems of divided attention could be resolved by adults adapting their signing (Spencer & Harris, 2006). For example, in order to make their signs visible to young infants, mothers may displace signs into a child's line of sight or onto the child's body or face (Harris, Clibbens, Chasin, & Tibbitts, 1989). With older infants, mothers may wait until the child looks up before they begin to sign. Strategies of this kind all help the child to make a link between ongoing events and the signs that accompany them.

One of the first examples we observed of an experienced, native signing, deaf mother adapting her signs was for the BSL sign LIGHT. This sign was produced in the context of a very familiar and often-repeated routine. The child would point up at a light on the ceiling in our laboratory and the mother would invariably sign LIGHT, holding her hand in the air so that it was between the child and the light (Clibbens & Harris, 1993), thus enabling the child to see both the sign and its referent. Other maternal signs had greater displacement. For example, the mother signed CAT on her child's face while they were looking at a picture of a cat in a book. Similar observation about maternal signing were made by Bencie Woll and Jim Kyle, who had also been considering the similarities and differences in the patterns of interaction between deaf mothers and their children and hearing mothers and their children (Woll & Kyle, 1989).

Maternal strategies that involve the adaptation of signs are very important for young infants. However, the adaptation of signs has its limitations, especially as infants develop into active toddlers. The displacement of signs from normal location into the child's line of sight and making signs on the child's face or body are only possible when child and adult are in close proximity; and such strategies become increasingly difficult to use as children become more mobile and are no longer content to sit on their mother's lap, or on the floor alongside her. Furthermore, only some signs can easily be displaced and, even where this is possible, important information carried on the signer's face is inevitably lost. Waiting to sign until a child pauses and looks up from an activity is potentially the most flexible strategy but it will only be successful if the child turns to look at the mother and, in particular, her face. An important development for young children who are learning to sign is to become aware of the signing channel of communication and thus to be attuned to the need to look up (Clibbens & Powell, 2003).

Because visual attention is so crucial for successful communication with deaf children, mothers who are deaf themselves – and thus very experienced at communicating with other people who are deaf – tend to be very proactive in gaining their young children's visual attention. (See Chapter 4 by Baker, this volume, for a further discussion of this point). Deaf mothers use a variety of strategies such as waving their hand in the child's line of sight, tapping the child on the arm or even banging on the floor so that vibrations carry across the room. Hearing parents of deaf children tend to use such strategies less often. Indeed, hearing parents are often less sensitive to the visual needs of a deaf child and find it more difficult to communicate in such a way that both the utterance and the surrounding nonverbal context to which it relates are simultaneously visible to the child (Harris, 2001; Harris & Mohay, 1997).

More recent research has confirmed our original finding that hearing mothers of deaf children often find it a challenge to initiate successful episodes of joint attention. Hearing mothers of deaf children, aged between 18 and 36 months, were found to have a success rate of 36% when they attempted to engage joint attention and this compared with a rate of almost 50% for hearing–hearing dyads (Nowakowski, Tasker, & Schmidt, 2009). This difference was statistically significant. Another analysis of interaction between mothers and their deaf two-year-olds directly compared joint attention in dyads where mothers were deaf with dyads where mothers were hearing (Gale & Schick, 2009). This comparison showed that deaf mothers were generally more responsive to their child's attentional focus and, in a 15-minute observation period, followed their child's attention an average of 11 times compared with 4.8 times for hearing mothers.

The Gale and Schick (2009) study also highlighted differences between the rhythm of interactions with a deaf child and similar interactions with a hearing child. In dyads where both mother and child were deaf, significantly less time was spent in symbol-infused joint attention (involving language) than in dyads where both partners were hearing. This was because the interactions in the deaf–deaf dyads were typically sequential whereas those of the hearing–hearing dyads were more commonly simultaneous. Hearing children were able to listen to their mother talking about objects and events in a shared focus of attention without needing to look at her whereas deaf children had to divide visual attention between the shared focus of attention and their mother. Interactions between deaf infants and their deaf mothers are characterised by pauses as mothers wait to gain their child attention and both mother and child are likely to produce fewer words than hearing children with hearing mothers (Harris et al., 1989; Harris & Mohay, 1997).

The study of developing patterns of visual attention has shown that there are other fundamental difference in the dynamics of successful interaction between deaf and hearing infants and their mothers. As already noted, deaf mothers with deaf children regularly elicit their attention through a variety of visual and tactile strategies, and this seems to be an essential aspect of successful communication with young deaf children (Spencer & Harris, 2006). Harris and Chasin (2005) compared deaf mothers of deaf children with hearing mother deaf-child dyads, deaf mother–hearing child dyads and hearing–hearing dyads. Deaf mothers of deaf children showed most attempts to elicit their children's attention but there was also evidence of elicitation in dyads where one partner was deaf and the other hearing. It was the dyads in which both partners were hearing that looked very different because hearing mothers of hearing children almost never elicited attention. The reason for this became clear in looking at what attracted the children's attention.

For hearing children, sound played a very important role in attracting attention to the mother and 70% of responsive looks (i.e., looks to the mother that were not the result of active elicitation) involved sound, either on its own or in conjunction with some action of the mother's. As you would expect, much of this sound was spoken language, and the sound of the mother's voice had a powerful effect on the hearing children, typically resulting in rapid attention to the mother. The attention-grabbing effect of speech and sound on hearing children explains why it is that hearing mothers of hearing children do not often need to elicit attention since, as soon as they begin to talk or make a sound, their child will typically turn to look at their face.

The Harris and Chasin study was published nearly 15 years ago and none of the children had been provided with a cochlear implant or digital hearing aid. As a result they had little or no access to sound, which meant that their mothers could not exploit the attention-directing properties of speech and other sounds. They had to make use of something else and this, most commonly, was movement.

However, a response to movement does not automatically bring attention to the face, as is the case with speech. Many of the mother's movements in the Harris and Chasin observations involved play objects. Mothers would often pick up a toy or book as they interacted with their child and this movement attracted the child's attention. Typically, if a child's attention was attracted in this way, it remained on the object being moved. Furthermore, the mother's intervention often provoked a negative reaction from the child, who would protest at the removal of the object and turn away from a potential interaction.

Prolonged focus on an object did not present a problem for hearing children. They were able to hear what their mother was saying while looking at a play object, and so be fully engaged in symbol-infused joint attention. However, the deaf mother of a deaf child had to find ways of getting her child's attention onto her face so she could communicate and, very often, mothers used physical strategies such as tapping, waving or banging to redirect attention to the face. The success of these strategies was evident in the fact that deaf children of deaf mothers looked to their mother's face as often as hearing children of hearing mothers (Harris & Chasin, 2005). However, children in both groups turned to look at their mother *less often* than children in the two groups where one partner was deaf and the other hearing. At first sight this may appear surprising because we might expect the best-attuned interactions to occur when mother and child have the same hearing status. However, the pattern of results can be understood when it becomes clear that a more extended interaction was likely to follow on from a look to the mother in the deaf–deaf and hearing–hearing dyads. This explanation is consistent with Spencer's (2000) finding that episodes of joint visual attention to the mother were of longer duration when the hearing status of mother and child was the same, and a more sophisticated linguistic exchange was likely to ensue. This finding was also supported by the more recent observations of Gale and Schick (2009).

Looking to the mother's face presents a different opportunity for communicating with deaf and hearing children. Having established an opportunity for a communicative opening, a hearing child can turn away and a conversation can continue. For deaf children, however, sustained looking at the mother is necessary. In a study of the development of looking behaviour in deaf infants between the age of 9 and 18 months of age (Chasin & Harris, 2008), deaf children of deaf mothers looked significantly longer at their mothers at 18 months than deaf children of hearing mothers. Across the age span, deaf children of deaf parents showed a higher proportion of looks to their mother's face than deaf children of hearing parents. The most likely explanation for these differences is that the children's looking behaviour had been shaped by the strategies used by mothers to engage attention. Deaf children of deaf mothers had become attuned to the communicative importance of the face at an earlier age than deaf children of hearing mothers.

The impact of cochlear implants on early communication

Since the first studies on interactions between deaf infants and toddlers and their parents were carried out there have been significant changes in the proportion of children with severe-profound hearing loss who now have access to spoken language and other sounds at an early age. This is because of the increasing availability of cochlear implants and digital hearing aids, coupled with universal newborn hearing screening and earlier diagnosis of hearing loss (See Chapter 1, this volume). As we saw in the previous section, the dynamics of early interaction are shaped, in part, by whether an infant has access only to visual information or access to both visual and auditory information. We might, therefore, expect that the technological advances for children with hearing loss will have an impact on the way that infants and caretakers interact and communicate.

There is now a growing body of evidence about the impact of early and effective hearing aid technology on infant–caretaker interaction and communication. The majority of these studies have focused on children who have received a cochlear implant and invariably they focus on hearing parents who, for the most part, use spoken language with their children and do not sign. Since the technology of implants continues to develop, and the age at which implant surgery takes place is falling, more recent studies provide the best evidence about how early interaction might be affected. One study (Tait, De Raeve, & Nikolopoulos, 2007) focused on a small group of children who had been implanted before the age of one year in the UK or Belgium. Recordings of their interaction with their hearing mother, or another familiar adult, were made shortly before implantation and at 6 and 12 months post-implant. The children were exposed to spoken language only and not to signing. The main analyses examined turn-taking by the infants, contrasting vocal and gestural turn-taking and comparing the total number of turns and proportions of each kind with the turns produced by a sample of hearing infants of similar age. Before implantation, the deaf infants produced fewer vocal turns than hearing children of the same age during the observation period and were much more likely to use gesture. The number of vocal turns was not significantly different 6 months after implantation. However, one year after implantation, the deaf children were again producing fewer vocal turns but more gestural turns than the hearing children – the same pattern that was evident before implantation – probably because the deaf children's spoken language had not developed to the same extent as their hearing peers. Tait et al. conclude that early cochlear implantation appears to change the way that deaf infants interact with their mothers but, at the same time, it has not removed differences between deaf and hearing children.

The Tait et al. (2007) study did not directly compare infants who had received a cochlear implant with those who had not. This comparison was made in a study of 26 hearing mothers with deaf toddlers, carried out in the United States (Tasker, Nowakowski, & Schmidt, 2010), 9 of whom had a cochlear implant and 17 of whom did not. (The two groups of deaf children were very similar and 4 of the children in the no-implant group had, in fact, received an implant that had not yet been activated.) Both sub-groups were compared with hearing toddlers of similar age, around 2 years. Both the span – number of communicative exchanges within an episode of joint attention – and quality of episodes of joint attention was greatest in the hearing–hearing dyads but the cochlear implant group showed longer spans and greater quality than the non-implant group. The mean age of implantation of children in this study was just under 17 months, so they had benefitted from early access to sound. Nevertheless, differences between deaf infants with cochlear implants and hearing infants remained.

This view that cochlear implants have changed the nature of early interaction, but have not yet succeeded in removing differences between deaf children with hearing mothers and hearing children, is supported by other studies. One study of toddlers with cochlear implants, carried out in Italy, looked at the language and conversational skills of 23 children whose cochlear implant had been activated around 14 months (Rinaldi, Baruffaldi, Burdos, & Caselli, 2013). The authors assessed the children's language, using the Italian version of the CDI (Caselli, Pasqualetti, & Stefanini, 2007). The CDI provides parents with a list of early spoken vocabulary and word combinations and asks them to tick all items that are understood or produced by their child. The children's pragmatic skills were evaluated using the Italian version of the Social Conversational Skills Rating Scale (Bonifacio & Girolametto, 2007). This is also a parental questionnaire and it asks about the child's ability to make requests and suggestions and to ask questions. It also asks about the child's responsiveness to questions and requests and ability to maintain turn-taking in conversation. Each of the measures was compared to normative data for hearing children.

The data on the vocabulary of the 23 children showed that 10 had scores that fell within normal range while 12 had scores that were more than one standard deviation below the mean (there were no data for one child whose parents did not complete the CDI). The data on word combinations showed a broadly similar pattern. The scores for social-conversation skills showed that all but one of the children, for whom normative data were available, had scores below the mean and only 3 children had scores within one standard deviation. As might be expected, there were significant correlations between vocabulary size and social-conversation skills.

The overall conclusion of the study was that many of the children were delayed in language development, in both vocabulary and grammar, but were even more delayed in their social-conversation skills. This highlights the continuing difficulties in early interaction experienced by young children with cochlear implants. It is also of note that there were no differences in the abilities of children who were implanted before 12 months and those who were implanted in the second year of life, suggesting that implanting before the age of 2 years is what appears to be important.

One final study sheds further light on the nature of joint attention and its relation to language development in young children with cochlear implants (Cejas, Barker, Quittner, & Niparko, 2014). This study, carried out in the United States, had 180 child participants with severe-profound hearing loss prior to cochlear implant surgery. All had hearing parents. They were assessed prior to implantation, and then every 6 months for the next 3 years, using a number of measures of interaction and language. The level of engagement of the infant was coded on an 8-point scale ranging from unengaged to symbol-infused joint attention. Language level was assessed using the American English version of the CDI (Fenson et al., 1994). The scores for the deaf children were compared with those of hearing children of similar age. The main findings were, first, that the language scores of the deaf children were significantly behind those of hearing children: none of the deaf children had language ages above 36 months whereas this was the case for just over 20% of the hearing children. Secondly, the level of joint attention was generally lower for the deaf children in that they spent more time engaged in lower levels of joint attention than their hearing peers. For example, among participants who were less than 18 months of age, the deaf children spent more time unengaged from the interaction and, for children aged between 18 and 36 months, the deaf group spent more time in onlooking – in which they passively observed their mother – and less time engaged in joint attention. Cejas et al. argue that the level of joint attention children were able to achieve was closely related to language age but not chronological age, since only language age was a significant predictor. This argument is consistent with the view that achieving a level of joint attention in which child and adult are mutually engaged with activities or objects and are able to converse about the ongoing events is key to acquiring language in the early stages.

What the four studies described in this section suggest is that the advent of early cochlear implantation has by no means resolved all of the inherent difficulties in interaction and communication for young deaf children of hearing parents. This conclusion naturally leads to the further question of what can be done to support early interaction so that deaf children of hearing parents can develop robust patterns of interaction that support language development. As Cejas et al. (2014, p. 1840) state at the conclusion of their article, '... parent-mediated interventions are urgently needed for families seeking cochlear implants for young deaf children'.

Interventions to support the development of joint attention

The provision of Universal Newborn Hearing Screening (UNHS) has provided an opportunity for hearing parents, who commonly have no experience of interacting with people who are deaf, to find out about how they can communicate effectively with their child and support the development of language. Inevitably the parents of an infant who has recently received a confirmatory diagnosis of hearing loss are confronted with huge quantities of information about the nature of their child's hearing loss, options for hearing aids, communication choices and educational possibilities and they can sometimes find this overwhelming. Interviews with service providers who saw parents after UNHS in Belgium (Matthijs et al., 2012) revealed that the advice and information provided was not consistent. For example, within the ENT department of hospitals, there was a very positive message about the benefits of cochlear implants and often no mention of the possibility of using sign language to communicate. Parents were typically advised to enrol their child in a mainstream school. Specialist teachers, on the other hand, were more likely to advocate beginning education in a school for the deaf – and using sign language – and then transferring to a mainstream setting. Across all service providers there was little discussion of ways in which parents could help their child to communicate.

There has been a very longstanding debate over the benefits of using sign language versus oral approaches with young deaf children (see Chapters 1, 8 and 10, this volume and Hall, 2017, for a recent commentary on this issue). The advent of cochlear implants and the consequent potential for children to benefit from additional auditory input has led to a resurgence of discussion in this area (Geers, Mitchell, Warner-Czyz, Wang, & Eisenberg, 2017). A recent paper argues that cochlear implants do not replace normal hearing and highlights the importance of early exposure to language, in a form which is accessible to the young child (Humphries et al., 2016). Research into the use of sign with children who receive a cochlear implant (Watson, Archbold, & Nikolopoulos, 2006; Watson, Hardie, Archbold, & Wheeler, 2008) shows that they tend to gradually rely less on signing and more on spoken language as time passes and their access to spoken language improves. These findings suggest that the early use of sign does not detract from the development of oral language and can, indeed, support it. However, some studies, including that of Geers et al. (2017), report findings that early sign language input provides no benefit over and above spoken language.

There is a clear need for further research before any such definitive statement can be made. For example, many of these studies do not distinguish between input based on natural and artificial signing and do not consider sign language in its broader cultural and communicative context (Hall, Schonstrom, & Spellum,

2017). This view is echoed in a recent paper by Matthijs and colleagues (Matthijs et al., 2017). They argue that there is a longstanding divide between a medical and a cultural-linguistic model when looking at potential early interventions and educational approaches for deaf children. The range of issues concerning the cultural and linguistic standing of signed versus spoken languages and the importance of achieving early access to language in a fully accessible form make it important not to jump to premature conclusions on the basis of studies considering a limited range of variables.

Providing parents with practical support to enable them to communicate effectively with their child and, in turn, to help their child to learn to communicate with them, has been the aim of a number of intervention programmes. One US study of 93 children who had received a cochlear implant attempted to identify effective strategies to promote language by analysing videos of parent–infant interactions prior to implant and over the following 3 years (Cruz, Quittner, Marker, & DesJardin, 2013). The parent–infant interactions involved both free and structured play and also problem-solving tasks in order to sample a range of different kinds of interaction. The main focus of the analysis was the nature and frequency of parental facilitative language techniques, which were divided into lower level techniques (e.g. imitating a child's utterance, asking a closed question or labelling an object) and higher level (e.g. asking an open-ended question, expanding a child's utterance or recasting an utterance into a question). These latter kinds of technique have been shown to support language development in hearing children with language delays and they have also been successfully taught to parents (Kaiser & Hancock, 2003). Cruz et al. found that the higher level techniques were associated with – and predicted – improvements in both the comprehension and production of spoken language, whereas there was no such relationship in the case of the lower level techniques. They argue that higher-level techniques provide children with a richer language experience that involved higher levels of joint attention.

These kinds of techniques are useful when children have begun to use and understand language. However, one of the most difficult things for parents of a deaf child is to provide opportunities for language learning in the very earliest stages when the child understands few words. Early provision of effective hearing aid technology has the potential to enable deaf infants to make use of sound in social interaction and so develop early vocabulary at a faster rate than before. A number of studies have shown that the early vocabulary of children with cochlear implants still lags behind that of hearing peers (Fagan, 2106) and, even though some of this delay can be accounted for by the difference between hearing age and chronological age (Fagan & Pisoni, 2010), it is clear that many young children with cochlear implants are not developing spoken language as quickly as might be hoped. In spite of the evidence of continuing delays, a review published a decade ago concluded that there was still little evidence about the effectiveness of early interventions to support language development in deaf children (Brown & Nott, 2006).

It is worth noting that it is difficult to develop effective interventions to support early language development even when children are hearing. A recent paper reports a randomised control trial of a language intervention for hearing 11-month olds from low SES families (McGillion, Pine, Herbert, & Matthews, 2017). The intervention was based on the strong line of evidence, mentioned earlier, that contingent talk embedded in joint attention is important for early language development. Families in the language intervention were shown a video that illustrated contingent talk and they were asked to practise it every day for a month. Caregiver communication was assessed at baseline and after 1 month of using contingent talk. Infant communication was assessed at baseline and then when the children were aged 12, 15, 18 and 24 months. When infants were 12 months old, caregivers who had been allocated to the language intervention group engaged in significantly more contingent talk than caregivers in the dental health control group. There was also evidence that their children produced significantly more words at 15 and 18 months than children in the control group. However, effects of the intervention did not persist at 24 months, which points to the need for interventions to be sustained over a long period.

One of the most long-standing interventions for young deaf children is that provided in Colorado (Yoshinaga-Itano, 2006, 2014), where universal newborn hearing screening began in 1992. While recognising the practical and ethical issues involved in evaluation of interventions, Yoshinaga-Itano argues that there is now good evidence to provide guidelines about key program components that promote positive outcomes. These include ensuring that familes who have a child who is deaf or hard-of-hearing have access to other, similar, families who can provide formal or informal support. She notes studies in which parents report participation in social networks with other parents of deaf children leads to less isolation, greater acceptance of their child, and improved interactional responsiveness from the child (Hintermair, 2000; Jackson, Wegner, & Turnbull, 2010). Yoshinaga-Itano also stresses the importance of hearing parents of deaf children having access to deaf individuals who can provide insights into specific issues about the nature of hearing loss. In the appendix of her review, she highlights key knowledge and skills that parents of deaf children should have to facilitate the development of language and communication. These include promoting the important role of caregivers in the development of communication skills, coaching parents in the use of strategies that promote a language rich learning environment, and assessing prelinguistic and early linguistic communication to ensure that development is progressing.

The research reviewed in this chapter suggests that, in the first two years of life, parents of deaf children need to ensure that they develop familiarity with routines, such as 'peekaboo' or building a tower and knocking it over, so that the children have a familiar social context in which to learn to understand their first words. Parents also need to ensure that children have access to the contingent language that accompanies the routines. In the case of spoken language, children need to learn to look at the face of the person who is speaking so that they can take advantage of information from movements of the lips and articulators (Kyle, MacSweeney, Mohammed, & Campbell, 2009). For some children, it may be appropriate to sign words at this early stage as well as saying them.

As children's language develops, parents can be encouraged to use strategies that build on what their child already knows and can say. This may involve elaborating something the child has said or asking open-ended questions. These are the same strategies that support language development in hearing children as they enlarge their vocabularies and learn how to construct sentences. Recent evidence about the language levels of deaf children suggests that, even with the wide availability of cochlear implants, many children with a severe-profound hearing loss enter primary school with a vocabulary level that is more than one year behind their chronological age (Harris, Terlektsi, & Kyle, 2017). This suggests that many deaf children will require additional support to develop a wide vocabulary – support that may be necessary through the early years of formal schooling.

References

Bakeman, R., & Adamson, L. B. (1984). Coordinating attention to people and objects in mother–infant and peer–infant interaction. *Child Development* 55(4), 1278–1289. https://doi.org/10.2307/1129997

Bonifacio, S., & Girolametto, L. (2007). *Questionario ASCB: Le abilita socio-converzationalidel bambino [ASCB questionnaire: Socio-conversational skills of the child]*. Tirrenia: Del Cerro.

Brown, P. M., & Nott, P. (2006). Family-centered practice in early intervention for oral language development: Philosophy, methods, and results. In P. E. Spencer & M. Marschark (Eds.), *Advances in the spoken language development of deaf and heard-of-hearing children* (pp. 136–165). New York, NY: Oxford University Press.

Bruner, J. S. (1975). The ontogenesis of speech acts. *Journal of Child Language* 2(1), 1–19. https://doi.org/10.1017/S0305000900000866

Bruner, J. S. (1983). The acquisition of pragmatic commitments In R. M. Golinkoff (Ed.), *The transition from prelinguistic to linguistic communication* (pp. 27–42). Hillsdale, NJ: Lawrence Erlbaum Associates.

Butterworth, G. E. (2001). Joint visual attention in infancy. In G. Bremner & A. Fogel (Eds.), *Blackwell handbook of infant development* (pp. 213–240). Malden, MA: Blackwell.

Carpenter, M., & Call, J. (2013). How joint is the joint attention of apes and human infants? In H. S. Terrace & J. Metcalfe (Eds.), *Agency and joint attention* (pp. 49–61). New York, NY: Oxford University Press. https://doi.org/10.1093/acprof:oso/9780199988341.003.0003

Caselli, M. C., Pasqualetti, P., & Stefanini, S. (2007). *Words and sentences in the first vocabulary of the child: New normative data from 18 to 36 months and short form of the questionnaire.* Milan: Franco Angeli.

Cejas, I., Barker, D. H., Quittner, A. L., & Niparko, J. K. (2014). Development of joint engagement in young deaf and hearing children: Effects of chronological age and language skills. *Journal of Speech, Language and Hearing Research* 57, 1831–1841. https://doi.org/10.1044/2014_JSLHR-L-13-0262

Chasin, J., & Harris, M. (2008). The development of visual attention in deaf children in relation to mother's hearing status. *Polish Psychological Bulletin* 3(1), 1–8. https://doi.org/10.2478/v10059-008-0001-z

Clibbens, J., & Harris, M. (1993). The acquisition of formational parameters in British Sign Language: A case study. In D. Messer & G. Turner (Eds.), *Critical influences on child language acquisition and development* (pp. 197–208). London: Macmillan. https://doi.org/10.1007/978-1-349-22608-5_10

Clibbens, J., & Powell, G. G. (2003). Joint attention and lexical development in typical and atypical communication. In S. von Tetzchner & N. Grove (Eds.), *Augmentative and alternative communication: Developmental issues* (pp. 28–37). London: Where.

Cruz, I., Quittner, A. L., Marker, C., & DesJardin, J. L. (2013). Identification of effective strategies to promote language in deaf children with cochlear implants *Child Development* 84(2), 543–549. https://doi.org/10.1111/j.1467-8624.2012.01863.x

Fagan, M. K. (2106). Spoken vocabulary development in deaf children with and without cochlear implants. In M. Marschark & P. E. Spencer (Eds.), *The oxford handbook of deaf studies in language* (pp. 132–145). New York, NY: Oxford University Press.

Fagan, M. K., & Pisoni, D. B. (2010). Hearing experience and receptive vocabulary development in deaf children with cochlear implants. *Journal of Deaf Studies and Deaf Education* 15(2), 149–161. https://doi.org/10.1093/deafed/enq001

Fenson, L., Dale, P., Resnick, S., Bates, E., Thal, D., & Pethick, S. J. (1994). Variability in early communicative development. *Monographs of the Society for Research in Child Development* 59(5), 1–73. https://doi.org/10.2307/1166093

Gale, E., & Schick, B. (2009). Symbol-infused joint attention and language use in mothers with deaf and hearing toddlers. *American Annals of the Deaf* 153(5), 484–503. https://doi.org/10.1353/aad.0.0066

Geers, A. E., Mitchell, C. M., Warner-Czyz, A., Wang, N.-Y., & Eisenberg, L. S. (2017). Early sign language exposure and cochlear implantation benefits. *Pediatrics.* https://doi.org/10.1542/peds.2016-3489

Hall, M. L., Schonstrom, K., & Spellum, A. (2017). Failure to distinguish among competing hypotheses. *Pediatrics.* Retrieved from <http://pediatrics.aappublications.org/content/early/2017/06/08/peds.2016-3489.comments>

Harris, M. (2001). It's all a matter of timing: Sign visibility and sign reference in deaf and hearing mothers of 18 month old children. *Journal of Deaf Studies and Deaf Education* 6, 177–185 https://doi.org/10.1093/deafed/6.3.177

Harris, M., Barlow-Brown, F., & Chasin, J. (1995). The emergence of referential understanding: Pointing and the comprehension of object names. *First Language* 15, 19–34. https://doi.org/10.1177/014272379501500101

Harris, M., & Chasin, J. (2005). Attentional patterns in deaf and hearing infants: The role of auditory cues. *Journal of Child Psychology and Psychiatry* 46, 1116–1123. https://doi.org/10.1111/j.1469-7610.2005.00405.x

Harris, M., Clibbens, J., Chasin, J., & Tibbitts, R. (1989). The social context of early sign language development. *First Language* 9, 81–97. https://doi.org/10.1177/014272378900902507

Harris, M., Jones, D., Brookes, S., & Grant, J. (1986). Relations between the non-verbal context of maternal speech and rate of language development. *British Journal of Developmental Psychology* 4, 261–268. https://doi.org/10.1111/j.2044-835X.1986.tb01017.x

Harris, M., & Mohay, H. (1997). Learning to look in the right place: A comparison of attentional behavior in deaf children with deaf and hearing mothers. *Journal of Deaf Studies and Deaf Education* 2, 95–103. https://doi.org/10.1093/oxfordjournals.deafed.a014316

Harris, M., Terlektsi, E., & Kyle, F. E. (2017). Literacy outcomes for primary school children who are deaf and hard of hearing: A cohort comparison study. *Journal of Speech, Language and Hearing Research* 60(3), 701–711. https://doi.org/10.1044/2016_JSLHR-H-15-0403

Hintermair, M. (2000). Hearing impairment, social networks, and coping: the need for families with hearing-impaired children to relate to to other parents and to hearing-impaired adults. *American Annals of the Deaf* 145(1), 41–53. https://doi.org/10.1353/aad.2012.0244

Humphries, T., Kushalnagar, P., Mathur, G., Napoli, D. J., Padden, C., Rathmann, C., & Smith, S. (2016). Language choices for deaf infants: Advice for parent regarding sign languages. *Clinical Pediatrics* 55(6), 513–517. https://doi.org/10.1177/0009922815616891

Jackson, C. W., Wegner, J. R., & Turnbull, A. P. (2010). Family quality of life following early identification of deafness. *Language, Speech and Hearing Services in Schools* 41(2), 194–205. https://doi.org/10.1044/0161-1461(2009/07-0093)

Kaiser, A. P., & Hancock, T. B. (2003). Teaching parents new skills to support thier youg children's development. *Infants & Young Children* 16(1), 9–21. https://doi.org/10.1097/00001163-200301000-00003

Kyle, F. E., MacSweeney, M., Mohammed, T., & Campbell, R. (2009). *The development of speechreading in deaf and hearing children: Introducing a new Test of Child Speechreading (ToCS).* Paper presented at the AVSP2009: International conferene on audio-visual speech processing, University of East Anglia, Norwich, UK.

Liszkowski, U., Carpenter, M., Henning, A., Striano, T., & Tomasello, M. (2004). Twelve-month-olds point to share attention and interest. *Developmental Science* 7, 297–307. https://doi.org/10.1111/j.1467-7687.2004.00349.x

Matthijs, L., Hardonk, S., Sermijn, J., Van Puyvelde, M., Leigh, G., Van Herreweghe, M., & Loots, G. (2017). Mothers of deaf children in the 21st century. Dynamic positioning between the medical and cultural–linguistic discourses *Journal of Deaf Studies and Deaf Education* 22(4), 365–377. https://doi.org/10.1093/deafed/enx021

Matthijs, L., Loots, G., Mouvet, K., Van Herreweghe, M., Hardonk, S., Van Hove, G., …Leigh, G. (2012). First information parents receive after UNHS detection of their baby's hearing loss. *Journal of Deaf Studies and Deaf Education* 17(4), 387–401. https://doi.org/10.1093/deafed/ens020

McGillion, M., Pine, J. M., Herbert, J. S., & Matthews, D. (2017). A randomised controlled trial to test the effect of promoting caregiver contingent talk on language development in infants from diverse socioeconomic status backgrounds. *Journal of Child Psychology and Psychiatry* 58, 1122–1131. https://doi.org/10.1111/jcpp.12725

Nowakowski, M. E., Tasker, S. L., & Schmidt, L. A. (2009). Establishment of joint attention in dyads involving hearing mothers of deaf children, and its relation to adaptive social behavior. *American Annals of the Deaf* 154(1), 15–29. https://doi.org/10.1353/aad.0.0071

Rinaldi, P., Baruffaldi, F., Burdos, S., & Caselli, M. C. (2013). Linguistic and pragmatic skills in toddlers with cochlear implant. *International journal of Language and Communication Disorders* 48(6), 715–725. https://doi.org/10.1111/1460-6984.12046

Scaife, M., & Bruner, J. S. (1975). The capacity for joint visual attention in the infant. *Nature* 253, 265–266. https://doi.org/10.1038/253265a0

Spencer, P. E. (2000). Looking without listening: Is audition a prerequisite for normal development of visual attention during infancy?. *Journal of Deaf Studies and Deaf Education* 5, 291–322. https://doi.org/10.1093/deafed/5.4.291

Spencer, P. E., & Harris, M. (2006). Patterns and effects of language input to deaf infants and toddlers from deaf and hearing mothers. In M. Marschark & P. E. Spencer (Eds.), *Sign language development* (pp. 71–101). Oxford: Oxford University Press.

Tait, M., De Raeve, L., & Nikolopoulos, T. P. (2007). Deaf children with cochlear implants before the age of 1 year: Comparison of preverbal communcation with normally hearing children. *International Journal of Pediatric Otorhinolaryngology* 71, 1605–1611. https://doi.org/10.1016/j.ijporl.2007.07.003

Tasker, S. L., Nowakowski, M. E., & Schmidt, L. A. (2010). Joint attention and social competence in deaf children with cochlear implants. *Journal of Developmental and Physical Disabilities* 22, 509–532. https://doi.org/10.1007/s10882-010-9189-x

Tomasello, M. (1995). Joint attention as social cognition In C. Moore & P. Dunham (Eds.), *Joint attention: Its origins and role in development* (pp. 103–130). Hillsdale, NJ: Lawrence Erlbaum Associates.

Watson, L. M., Archbold, S. M., & Nikolopoulos, T. (2006). Children's communication code five years after cochlear implantation: Changes over time according to age at implant. *Cochlear Implants International* 7(2), 77–91. https://doi.org/10.1179/146701006807508061

Watson, L. M., Hardie, T., Archbold, S. M., & Wheeler, A. (2008). Parents' views on changing communication mode after cochlear implantation. *Journal of Deaf Studies and Deaf Education* 13, 104–116. https://doi.org/10.1093/deafed/enm036

Woll, B., & Kyle, J. G. (1989). Communication and language development in children of deaf parents. In S. von Tetzchner, L. S. Siegel, & L. Smith (Eds.), *The social and cognitive aspects of normal and atypical language development*. New York, NY: Springer. https://doi.org/10.1007/978-1-4612-3580-4_7

Woolfe, T., Herman, R., Roy, P., & Woll, B. (2010). Early vocabulary development in deaf native signers: A British Sign Language adaptation of the communicative development inventories. *Journal of Child Psychology and Psychiatry* 51(3), 322–331. https://doi.org/10.1111/j.1469-7610.2009.02151.x

Yoshinaga-Itano, C. (2006). Early identification, communication modality, and the development of speech and spoken language skills: Patterns and considerations. In P. E. Spencer & M. Marschark (Eds.), *Advances in the spoken language development of deaf and heard-of-hearing children* (pp. 298–327). New York NY: Oxford University Press.

Yoshinaga-Itano, C. (2014). Principles and guidelines for early intervention after confirmation that a child is deaf or hard of hearing. *Journal of Deaf Studies and Deaf Education* 19(2), 143–175. https://doi.org/10.1093/deafed/ent043

CHAPTER 3

Overlap in turn-taking in signed mother–child dyadic and triadic interactions

Anne Baker and Beppie Van den Bogaerde

Little is known about the development of the rules of turn-taking when signing, such as the extent to which overlap is allowed and when, and which attention strategies are used by signers when overlapping. This topic was investigated by comparing the more complex triadic situation (involving three people) of a deaf mother and her two deaf twins aged 5;6 years, together with how the adult communicated with these two children individually. Visual attention for the beginning of utterances was mostly established, but more so in the dyadic than the triadic situation. Seating position appeared to be relevant. More explicit strategies to attract eye-gaze were used in the triadic than the dyadic situation, including less usual strategies. Despite the conversation being between three people and needing checks with all participants, there was not more overlap in the triadic situation. Development in turn-taking is clearly still continuing after age six years.

1. Introduction[1]

Little work exists on turn-taking in signed interaction – few studies have been carried out on adult communication and even fewer on adult–child interaction. A small number of studies on adult turn-taking systems in American Sign Language

---

1. The collaboration between Bencie and us goes back a long way – to 1988 – but Bencie has been an inspiration to our field for far longer. She started off in the domain of language acquisition (Woll, 1978) and this interest has remained throughout her sign linguistics career, during which she has considered many aspects of sign language acquisition.

Bencie was also in the PhD committee for Beppie, who disappointed her by – at the last minute – removing part of the dissertation about which Bencie wanted to question her. Bencie improvised by asking a question about transcription – which resulted, some years later, in our collaborative book on methods and procedures in sign language acquisition studies (Baker, Van den Bogaerde, & Woll, 2009). Our chapter here is not on a subject that Bencie studied herself but includes her work as a baseline for our assumptions and research.

https://doi.org/10.1075/tilar.25.03bak
© 2020 John Benjamins Publishing Company

(ASL, Baker, 1977), British Sign Language (BSL, Coates & Sutton-Spence, 2001) and Brazilian Sign Language (LIBRAS, McLeary & Leite, 2012) have described the role of overlap occurring in conversations, as well as the existence of modality-specific attention-getting strategies to gain or hold a turn (see Harris & Clibbens, Chapter 2). One dominant aspect in sign language turn-taking is eye-gaze. It is of course crucial that the conversation partner sees the signer's communication. The start of utterances is important since the addressee can be informed about the status of the information being signed. Background (or old) information is usually provided first in the utterance in many signed languages (Kimmelman & Pfau, 2016). But sometimes new information is highlighted. In addition, making eye-contact (mutual eye-gaze) can be used to indicate the signer's willingness to hand over the turn. Checking for eye-gaze to fulfil these pragmatic functions can be very complex in turn-taking in signed multi-person conversations.

All children need to learn the pragmatic rules for interaction (e.g., Galloway & Richards, 1994; Casillas, 2014; Filipi, 2014) and research in spoken languages indicate that various aspects are still being learned after the age of three years (Casillas, Bobb & Clark, 2016). Pragmatic skills comprise turn-taking competencies, including such aspects as asking questions, initiating topics, expanding and clarifying unclear utterances, and sustaining conversational episodes (Cekaite, 2013). Cekaite emphases that achieving adult-like conversational coherence and improving topical relatedness in conversations continues throughout adolescence (cf. 2013, p. 3)

Children being raised with a sign language need also to learn the cultural and language rules of turn-taking, master eye-gaze behaviour, learn the rules for overlap and develop the social and cognitive skills for getting appropriate attention, realising that attention is shared, and learning polite behaviour. It is not clear how long the development of these pragmatic aspects of sign language interaction takes (Prinz & Prinz, 1985; Van den Bogaerde, 2000; Baker & Van den Bogaerde, 2012). Because of the complexity of sharing visual attention between the signer and the object being talked about, it is to be expected, for example, that children will take longer to master the eye-gaze rules in a sign language. But on the whole, based on studies on pragmatic development in spoken languages (e.g. Cekaite, 2013), we may assume that sign language pragmatic skills too will continue to develop well into adolescence.

This chapter aims to contribute to the body of knowledge on pragmatic development in deaf children using a sign language. The turn-taking behaviour of two deaf twins in interaction with their Deaf mother, once in a dyadic setting and once in a triadic play situation will be studied. Thus, the dimension of multi-party interaction will be added to previous results from the literature.

2. Turn-taking

The ability to organize verbal interaction by taking turns involves selecting the appropriate place for a verbal contribution in conversation. Rules that govern turn-taking, both in spoken and in sign languages, seem to be driven by universal aspects and cultural or language-specific features. Stivers et al. (2009) tested these two opposing hypotheses:

    i.   a universal system hypothesis, by which turn-taking is a universal system with minimal cultural variability, and

    ii. a cultural variability hypothesis, by which turn-taking is language and culture dependent.

The universal system hypothesis in (i) predicts a unimodal distribution of turn transitions with most transitions occurring with as good as no overlap in all languages, whereas the cultural variability hypothesis (ii) predicts that overlap is more common in some languages and gaps more common in others.

(Stivers et al., 2009: 10587)

Stivers et al. (2009) looked at the distribution of turn transitions (between polar questions and answers), and the role of eye-gaze in ten typologically different languages from diverse cultures across the five continents. They found substantial support for the universal system hypothesis, with minimal overlap and minimal gap between turns appearing to be the target. They did observe cultural differences between the languages but interpret these as not implying fundamentally different types of turn-taking mechanisms. Stivers et al. (2009) summarize the role of eye-gaze in turn-taking from the literature as follows:

Research on conversation in European languages suggests that a speaker's gaze toward a listener may increase the pressure to respond and to respond quickly: eye gaze does this by indicating who is addressed, by providing early possible cues that the speaker's turn is now coming to an end and signalling the speaker's heightened expectancy for a response. (Stivers et al., 2009, 10588)

Eye-gaze directed at an addressee during the formulation of a question appeared to elicit faster responses, but the authors found measurable cultural variation here. Nevertheless, they conclude that the differences found, such as a mean of a quarter of a second in the mean offset of each turn, do not warrant a conclusion that the turn-taking systems are fundamentally different. Therefore, if turn-taking behaviour follows a common path in spoken languages (i.e., the addressee responds more quickly when the speaker is looking at him/her), the same systems can be expected to also apply to signed languages.

Coates and Sutton-Spence (2001) studied the informal interaction in British Sign Language (BSL) in two groups of deaf friends, one group consisting of four females, the other of four males. Besides finding many instances of 'one at a time talk' (p. 525), there was a considerable amount of overlap. They concluded that overlap occurs primarily for establishing the collaborative floor amongst the friends; that is, for giving simultaneous feedback about the topic by using strategies such as repetition for clarification. McLeary and Leite (2012) described how, in a dyadic situation in Brazilian Sign Language (LIBRAS), their two deaf participants adhered mainly to the 'one-party-at-the-time' rule (Schegloff, 2000, p. 2). However, in such a face-to-face conversation, other elements than linguistic cues are also relevant, such as body-movements, gestures, or events in the near surroundings (e.g., a telephone flashing). These should all be taken into account. The visual-manual modality in which sign languages are perceived and produced also plays a role. For instance, De Vos, Torreira and Levinson (2015) described how turn overlaps are more frequent in Sign Language of the Netherlands (NGT) than in many spoken languages and suggest that the increased amount of overlap may be a consequence of having larger and slower articulators.

Children learning spoken languages are initially slower in their turn-taking behaviour than adults (Casillas, Bobb, & Clark, 2016); it is suggested that this is due to developing linguistic processing and production planning as well as social-cultural rule-learning. For example, in order to take a turn quickly and not risk another person seizing the turn, the addressee needs to predict when an utterance is going to be completed and thus when a turn taking chance will be offered. This requires linguistic ability and also fast processing (Levinson & Torreira, 2015). It is also necessary to have insight into what other people may be thinking and feeling, a *Theory of Mind* (e.g. Woolfe, Want, & Siegal, 2003). Overlap in turns can be allowed, but is restrained by conversational rules, which vary according to the linguistic community. Cekaite (2013) showed that the development of turn-taking skills is quite protracted, continuing up to at least 11 years. The author describes turn taking procedures as 'situationally and culturally sensitive, varying depending on participation frameworks (dyadic or multiparty), activities, and social settings'. The time-line of development of turn-taking based on previous research is based on Western societies, where children are treated as conversational partners from very early on and is therefore relative. As such, turn-taking begins to develop long before children produce language themselves. By age three children manage their interactions in peer groups, following rules but usually taking longer than adults between turns. Such children, often practice multi-party interactions during family meal times or in kindergarten settings, but turn-taking management takes much longer in these contexts. In her review Casillas (2014) mentions that children do not usually learn how to claim a turn in multi-party conversations before the age of six years.

In instruments measuring social interaction[2] it is usually expected that children will start to take turns in games such as peek-a-boo by one year, will share attention between objects and the adult by 18 months, can take a turn in a conversation by 3 years, and can take turns in multi-party conversation between 5 and 11 years. The question then is how children acquire appropriate turn-taking behaviour in signed languages, in accordance to the cultural and linguistic rules of their community, in dyadic and triadic or multi-party conversations.

An obvious prerequisite for sign language interaction is that visual attention needs to be procured by the signer from the addressee(s) (e.g., Wilbur & Petitto, 1983/2009). Appropriate visual attention and eye-gaze behaviour in turn-taking are important features that need to be acquired by young children (Harris et al., 1989; Roos, Cramér-Wolrath, & Falman, 2016; Sutton Spence & Woll, 1999; Van den Bogaerde, 2000). The studies show that this process takes several years. (See also Chapter 2 in this volume on this topic by Harris & Clibbens and Chapter 8 by Dye & Robinson on visual attention development, also this volume).

Deaf adults obtain attention for a turn by using explicit attentional strategies, such as waving the hand or tapping someone lightly on shoulder or arm, but they also use implicit strategies such as waiting for eye contact before starting to sign, or by simply starting to sign and expecting their interlocutor to perceive the movement and direct their eye-gaze toward the signer. Turns (in a dyadic situation using sign language) are usually maintained or held by avoiding eye-contact by averting the eyes from the addressee(s) while signing. Baker (1977) described how signers, when beginning a statement, usually do not look at the addressee (−Gaze), but when asking a question, they usually do (+Gaze). Likewise, addressees can indicate that the signer may initiate a turn by (+Gaze), or maintain their own inactivity (i.e. by not signing). An indication that the signer is willing to yield the floor to the addressee is by returning his/her gaze. Supposedly, when there is more than one interlocutor, the person who is looked at at the end of a signer's turn is the one to whom the floor is given. Eye-gaze direction thus serves a very important role in turn allocation and turn management in situations with more than two conversation partners (Van Herreweghe, 2002).

The study of twins in interaction is fairly rare and is usually not used as an explicit methodology as is the case of our study. Studying twins does, however, have some implications. Rendle-Short, Skelt, and Rambley (2015) studied the interaction between a hearing mother with her four-year-old twins (both hearing boys) in English. This situation had also been studied earlier by Tomasello,

---

2. For example the Humber Social Communication Development Milestones: <https://www. humber.nhs.uk/Downloads/Services/Childrens%20therapies/SLT/Milestones/Social%20 Communication%20%20Developmental%20Milestones%20Final.pdf>

Manle, and Kruger (1986). A study of twins has the advantage that both children are of the same age and have the same close relation with the adult. Rendle-Short et al. (2015) conclude that twins are more frequently in a triadic situation (three persons involved[3]) and may therefore learn multi-party turn-taking skills slightly earlier than children who do not have this practice. They found that the hearing mother used eye-gaze to regulate the attention of the hearing children and the conversation, and that the twins constantly monitored the ongoing interaction so that they could appropriately time their own contributions to the conversation (Rendle-Short et al., 2015, p. 79). The mother also used a child's name or asked a question to gain attention. Eye-gaze, besides content of talk, gestures and body posture, is clearly important in the interaction with this mother and her twins in a spoken language since it is a multi-party conversation. It raises the question how more important this may be in a signed multi-party conversation.

By studying the characteristics of turn-taking behaviour of the twins in our study in both a dyadic and a triadic interaction with their mother, we hope to gain more insights into various aspects of turn-taking in children. We formulated the following research questions:

1. Is visual attention to signing established at the beginning of utterances by the children and their mother?
2. What attentional strategies are used by the children and their mother?
3. How much overlap in turn-taking is found in the children and their mother?
4. Are there differences between the dyadic and triadic situation in these three aspects?

In the next section we will describe the methodology, followed by the results. In the final section we will give our conclusions and discuss the implications for turn-taking development in sign language interaction.

Methodology

The purpose of this study was to investigate the characteristics of turn-taking in dyadic mother–child interactions and to compare these with turn-taking in triadic interactions. This was done in the form of a case study of two children in the same family with the same parent at the same age.

The participants in this study were two deaf children (Laura and Mark) in interaction with the same deaf mother. The children are twins so that age is not a

---

3. In other literature the term 'triadic' is used to refer to two people interacting with the environment (see Chapter 2, Harris & Clibbens). Here we will use the term to refer to three people in interaction.

significant variable when considering any differences between the two children, although of course there may be individual variation between any two children of the same age. The twins have an older hearing sibling and their father is a *coda*, a hearing child of deaf parents. NGT was used consistently in family interactions, but also some spoken Dutch and both languages in combination. The mother and the three children had been regularly filmed as part of a longitudinal sign language acquisition project (see Baker & Van den Bogaerde, 2008; Van den Bogaerde, 2000; Van den Bogaerde & Baker, 2002, 2006).[4] They were recorded in spontaneous interaction situations (see Figure 1).

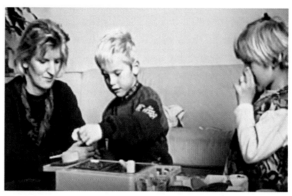

Figure 1. The triadic play situation with the deaf mother and twins at age 5;6.

The data for the analyses of this study were taken from recordings made with each of the twins with their mother in a dyadic situation at age 6;0. The data for the triadic situation were obtained from a recording made at age 5;6. The timespan of only six months between the two situations, as well as the different setting, do not warrant a developmental analysis. Five minutes of interaction were analysed from each recording; these five minutes did not fall within the first five minutes of the recording so that all participants had relaxed into the situation. The family was used to the recording situation; the camera person was a hearing fluent signer. The utterances produced during the interaction were transcribed and annotated in ELAN.[5] Utterances such as 'yes' (head nod), 'no' (head shake), and interactive gestures like 'shrug' were excluded.

---

4. This project ran at the University of Amsterdam and collected data from three deaf children and three hearing children in deaf families from 1988 to 1997. These data are available for further analyses from the Max Planck Institute Nijmegen on application.

5. ELAN is open source software used for the Language Archive at the Max Planck Institute Nijmegen:<https://tla.mpi.nl/tools/tla-tools/elan/>

In order to answer the question whether visual attention to signing had been established at the beginning of utterances for each participant, each utterance was analysed with respect to the behaviour of the addressee(s). The direction of eye-gaze of the addressee(s) was noted at the beginning of the signer's utterance. In the case of the triadic interaction both addressees were scored separately. This resulted in a binary score for each addressee: visual attention yes or attention no.

As discussed above, the signer could use different strategies to obtain visual attention for the communication from the addressee(s), such as explicit hand waving or tapping, implicit waiting for eye contact, or shifting the signing space into the visual field of the addressee(s). Each utterance was analysed using a binary coding with respect to the type of strategy used by the signer (explicit or implicit).[6]

As noted in the introduction, overlap in adult–adult signing is common. Each utterance was coded for overlap and thus the percentages of utterances with overlap reflect the amount of overlap in the whole conversation. The overlaps were further sub-coded. An interruption was noted if the signer stopped as a result of the overlap. The interrupting participant was noted, and the proportions of these calculated as a percentage of the other participant's utterances. The overlaps could also be simultaneous starts (percentage of all utterances). Our main focus was on the interruptions from the child, since children in general have been found to master the ability to break into ongoing conversation just before age 6;0 (Casillas, 2014: 55).

As stated earlier, the analyses also indicated whether the dyadic and triadic situations function differently in these three aspects (visual attention established at utterance start, attention strategy used, and overlap). The scores were therefore compared between the two situations. That is, we determined whether each participant behaved differently in the two situations. The analysis was purely qualitative and we did not compare situations statistically. We expected there to be more overlap in the triadic situation, mostly by the children, since multi-person conversations are more complex and thus more difficult to manage than dyadic ones.

It was also possible to compare the results partially with an earlier study in which the same two deaf children had been followed at a younger age, at 2;0 and 3;0. Mark has also been compared earlier with his hearing brother Jonas at the same age of 6;0. These analyses, reported in Van den Bogaerde and Baker (2014), focussed on the differences in the turn-taking behaviour of a deaf child compared to a signing hearing child.

---

6. Since the turns consisted almost exclusively of one utterance, the utterances were also at the beginning of the turn.

Results

In order to give a general picture of the amount of participation in the conversation as a background measure, the percentage of utterances produced by each participant was calculated (see Table 1). Barton and Tomasello (1991) found in their research that there is most often a balance between parent and young child, although the parent is usually slightly more dominant in conversation with younger children.

Table 1. Percentage of utterances produced by each participant in each situation

Situation	Mother	Mark	Laura
Dyadic Mark n = 186	56	44	–
Dyadic Laura n = 148	67	–	33
Triadic n = 128	48	22	30

The mother was dominant in all three situations although she contributed less in the dyadic conversation with Mark than with Laura and least in the triadic conversation. This level of participation by the child was very similar to his hearing brother at the same age (Van den Bogaerde & Baker, 2014). Mark had slightly less participation in the triadic conversation compared to his sister. In general, the interaction seems to follow the general pattern expected at this age.

As discussed earlier, it is important to visually attend to signing in order to participate fully in a conversation. The person who wishes to take a turn may wait for eye-gaze from the addressee(s) before starting to sign. Participants may also regularly check back with the other participant(s) to see if they are signing. The percentage of utterances produced by each signer was calculated in terms of whether the beginning of the utterance was seen by the addressee(s) (Figure 2).

Clearly from Figure 2 the dyadic situation is much easier for interlocutors to capture the beginning of the utterances. Both children at this age see the vast majority of their mother's communications. From the analysis done in Van den Bogaerde and Baker (2014) it was clear that the percentage of utterances seen by Mark increased considerably over time: from 77% at age 2;0 to 91% at age 3;0 up to 98% at age 6;0; this was higher than for the hearing brother Jonas (around 62%). He also had access to his mother's utterances because she also used her voice occasionally, to which he had aural access. He looked less often at his mother compared to his deaf brother.

Despite the children's high level of ability in the dyadic situation, they saw far fewer utterances in the triadic situation, both from the mother and from each other: 46% (Laura) and 36% (Mark). Mark saw less of the communication than

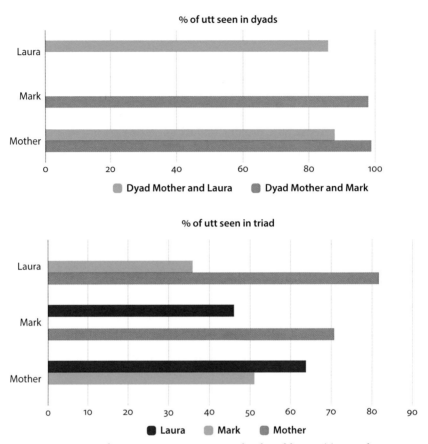

Figure 2. Percentage of utterances per signer seen by the addressee(s) in each situation

his sister, which might be related to his production of slightly fewer utterances in this context (see Figure 2). This could also be due to his sitting position between his mother and sister.[7] He has to look both right and left to catch utterances from the others, whereas both his mother and Laura could see the other two at the same time from their positions (see Figure 1).

Attention can be obtained for initiating signed utterances using either explicit strategies, such as hand waving, or implicit strategies, such as waiting for eye-gaze towards the signer. If no explicit strategy is used, then the strategy used is by definition implicit.

Deriving the percentage of implicit strategies from Figure 3, it is obvious that implicit strategies are far more common attention getters across interlocutors.

---

7. We thank those present at the University of Connecticut's (Storrs, USA) presentation of this research, by invitation of Diane Lillo-Martin in October 2016, for pointing this out to the authors.

Previous research has established that this is a preference in signing children from as early as the second year (Harris et al., 1989; Van den Bogaerde, 2000). Figure 3 also shows that in the dyadic conversation both Laura and her mother used more explicit strategies than in the dyadic conversation with Mark. This was possibly influenced by the form of the conversation (Baker et al., 2009), since Laura and her mother were looking at photographs part of the time and so their visual attention was on the pictures. This situation occurs regularly in many literate families but requires considerable skill in dividing attention between the text and pictures and the conversation partner (Bacchini, Kuiken, & Schoonen, 1995). Interestingly, in the dyadic conversation with Jonas (hearing) (Van den Bogaerde & Baker, 2014), the mother used her voice as an explicit strategy to gain his attention. This does not occur in the deaf–deaf interactions.

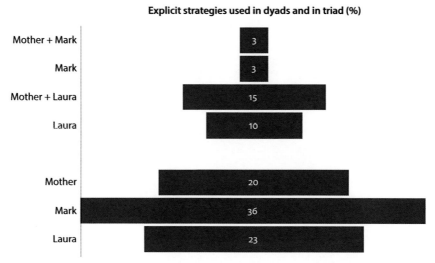

Figure 3. Percentage of use of explicit attention strategies per utterance per signer in each situation

The percentage of explicit strategies used was considerably higher for all participants in the triadic conversation (Figure 3), although particularly for the children. It is essentially more difficult to gain the attention of two addressees compared to one using implicit strategies. The mother used tapping or hand waving. The children, however, at this age of 5;6, used a different range of strategies that are not generally acceptable in adult–adult interaction. They held the arm of an addressee or held the hands of the last signer (Figure 4) in order to claim the turn. They signed very close to the face of one of the addressees (Figure 5) or used their elbow to give the other a dig in the ribs. These may be manifestations of informal attention strategies that occur between family members or people that are very familiar with one another, but are not part of the more formal system for taking turns. Casillas (2014, p. 55) also describes tugging at hems, turning a caregiver's face or repeatedly *calling* attention to themselves as examples in spoken interaction.

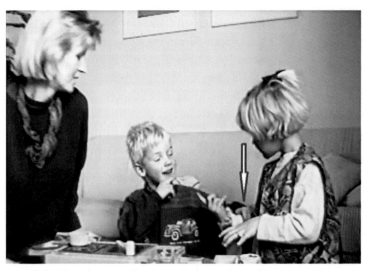

Figure 4. Mark holding the arm of Laura in order to claim the turn

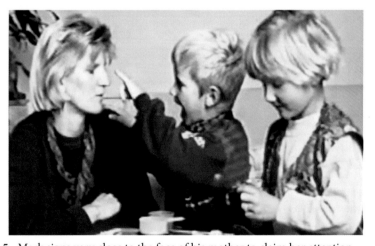

Figure 5. Mark signs very close to the face of his mother to claim her attention

Mark was less successful in gaining attention than Laura. Possibly his position between his mother and his sister was less favourable for gaining attention.

The little previous research that has been done on adult–adult sign interaction has indicated a considerable amount of overlap in conversations, which can be related to floor sharing (Coates & Sutton-Spence, 2001). The percentage of utterances with overlapping signing was calculated per situation (Table 2).

Table 2. Percentage of utterances with overlapping signing in each situation

Situation	% Utterances with overlapping signing
Dyadic Mark	63
Dyadic Laura	20
Triadic	33

It is striking that the conversation between Mark and his mother produced the most overlap. This was not apparently related to one not seeing the signing of the other, since the percentages of seen utterances in that dyad were high (see Table 2). Interestingly, in the dyadic situation Mark and his mother had a very fluent conversation, and apparently simultaneous signing did not hinder reciprocal understanding. Laura, on the other hand, was more reluctant to engage and was more hesitant before taking her turn. She and her mother were also part of the time looking at photographs and so attention had to be switched from the picture to the communication. This may explain why there was less overlap in this conversation, possibly because it takes longer to coordinate mutual eye gaze, checking attention to the pictures and signing in this situation.

It might be expected that the triadic situation would produce the most overlap, but this was not the case. One form of overlap is when both conversation partners simultaneously start to sign. This was measured as a percentage of all turns (Table 3). In the triadic conversation the simultaneous starts were measured for each of the children in terms of the simultaneous starts they were involved in.

Table 3. Percentage of simultaneous starts in each situation

Situation	Mark	Laura
Dyadic with Mark	17	–
Dyadic with Laura	–	1
Triadic	11	13

Laura had far fewer simultaneous starts in the dyadic conversation, Mark had more, but on the whole simultaneous starts do not occur a great deal. It is not clear why the differences occur. It is possible to conjecture that Mark is more focussed on signing himself but there is no independent evidence of this. The longitudinal data in Van den Bogaerde and Baker (2014) do not indicate a developmental pattern: the numbers of these simultaneous starts between 2;0 and 6;0 are quite low.

It was not expected that the mother would often interrupt the children and this was in fact the case. Table 4 presents therefore the frequency of interruptions made by the children; in the triadic situation the child can interrupt either the mother or their sibling. The frequency is expressed as a percentage of the utterances by the other participant(s).

Table 4. Percentage of interruptions made by the child participants in each situation

Situation	Mark	Laura
Dyadic: Mark interrupts	43	–
Dyadic: Laura interrupts	–	30
Triadic:	39	36

Mark interrupted slightly more than Laura in their dyadic conversations, but in the triadic situation there was no difference between the two children. From the longitudinal data in Van den Bogaerde and Baker (2014) there was no clear developmental pattern in either Mark or his hearing brother, Jonas. However, both children showed a dip at age 3;0 (28% and 14% respectively), which possibly reflects a beginning in awareness of not signing simultaneously at that age. The increase at age 6;0 may then be interpreted as a growing ability to sign in the context of a collaborative floor. This suggestion requires more research to evaluate, but would tie in neatly with the development of Theory of Mind, as mentioned earlier, which is starting around age 4;0 (see for example Woolfe et al., 2003).

Discussion and conclusion

Children, whether speaking or signing, need to acquire complex combinations of conversational skills such as turn-taking procedures, ability to initiate topics, the understanding of how to make their interjections relevant, and the ability to recognize and repair breakdowns in mutual communication (Cekaite, 2013, pp. 2–4). As mentioned earlier, these conversational skills are also closely connected to their cognitive and social development (e.g., Peters, n.d.). For hearing children a strong connection between Executive Functions (EF) and pragmatic skills was found for children aged 3;10–5;7 by Blain-Brière, Bouchard and Bigras (2014), although they did not consider turn-taking explicitly. We know a little about the development of Theory of Mind in deaf signing children (e.g., Woolfe et al., 2003; Schick, De Villiers, De Villiers, & Hoffmeister, 2007). There is a report of some delay in deaf children with hearing parents but deaf children of deaf parents have no delay in first order false-belief tasks. In a study of EF in signing deaf children of deaf parents no delay was found in the EF aspects studied (Kotowicz et al., 2017). However, the link between Theory of Mind, EF, and pragmatic abilities has not been studied in these populations.

As we discussed earlier, in signed interactions it is highly important for visual attention to the signing to be established at the beginning of the utterances. Children have to learn to watch for communication and then pay appropriate attention in time to perceive the content of the utterances. These capacities are closely connected to underlying executive function skills and meta-pragmatic skills like knowing when and how to talk/sign and providing contingent utterances. Our results have shown that the children are seeing a large majority of the beginning of the mother's utterances in the dyadic situation at age 6;0. This was expected on the basis of earlier research which showed that this was being achieved in dyads around age three (Van den Bogaerde, 2000). In the triadic conversation, however, the children especially found it more difficult to pay visual attention to the person signing. The mother was more successful but did better in the dyad settings. Mark has the most difficulty to catch the beginning of utterances, perhaps because he was seated in the middle position.[8] He had to take time to swivel his head to catch communication and thus missed more.

Since the mother was far more successful in perceiving the language of her child conversation partners, this suggests that considerable development will take place after the age of six years. This fits in with the time-line as described for hearing children in spoken conversations (Casillas, 2014). There is still a need for more adult–adult conversation analysis; when the adult level will be achieved also has to be established by future research.

In the dyadic conversations implicit attentional strategies are predominantly used; that is, the signer waits for eye contact or starts signing with the expectation that the conversational partner will look. Children have to learn these implicit strategies specific to the signing situation. They are, however, an example of the interactive alignment, as discussed in general with respect to all conversations, whether signed or spoken. Garrod and Pickering (2009) discussed how conversations are joint actions involving alignment in terms of both language and non-linguistic behaviours. They argued that alignment involves prediction in both comprehension and production. In signing situations, for example, the child needs to learn that starting to sign in the periphery of the addressee's visual field will lead to visual attention.

Because of the greater complexity of checking two other people for communication in the triadic situation, explicit strategies are more common in all participants. The explicit strategies take the form of tapping or waving, which have also been observed in adult–adult interaction in many sign languages (Baker, 1977).

---

8. The seating arrangement was influenced by this being a play situation and a camera being present. Under other circumstances it could be said that choosing your seating position in a sign conversation is reflection of your awareness of the conditions needed for good turn-taking.

The children, however, also use quite invasive strategies, such as signing directly in front of the partner's face, holding the arm of the other to stop them signing, or elbowing each other. Once Laura even hit her brother quite hard in the chest with her fist to get his attention (Figure 6).

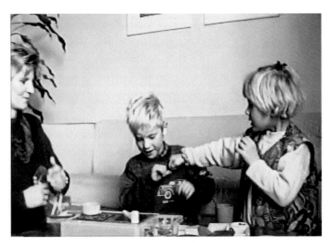

Figure 6. Laura punches Mark on the chest to get the turn

These strategies do not seem to be part of formal interaction in NGT, but it is as yet unknown if such strategies are used amongst signing adults who know each other well in informal situations. We do not yet know specifically what the politeness conventions are for different sign languages, although Hoza (2007) has described them for ASL. We also do not know when they are acquired by deaf children of deaf parents.

Overlap has been observed in most adult signed interaction, mainly with the function of creating a collaborative floor (Coates & Sutton Spence, 2001). In the first two years of life children overlap because they have not yet learned the rules of alternate turn-taking. They seem to become aware of not overlapping around the age of three years. Children then have to learn when overlap is conversationally and culturally acceptable (e.g., Peters, n.d.; Casillas, 2014), such when giving feedback and creating consensus. The conversations in the current study show different amounts of overlap in different settings. Mark's dyadic conversation with his mother runs very smoothly and this conversation has the greatest amount of overlap. The dyadic conversation with Laura ran less smoothly since she was less motivated to communicate; they were also looking at photographs requiring more use of explicit attentional strategies to ensure their signing was seen. The triadic conversation did not show a greater amount of overlap, which may be related to the need for more explicit attentional strategies. Mark appears to interrupt more than Laura in the triadic conversation. Inspection indicated that his use of explicit attentional strategies was not always successful. These two aspects are likely to be related.

This study suggests that the triadic conversation situation has an influence on turn-taking. This type of turn-taking requires more explicit attentional strategies to ensure that conversational contributions are seen. The children at age six years have not yet reached an adult level in controlling this dynamic. Clearly considerable development still has to take place. Research with spoken language acquisition indicates that the fine tuning of turn-taking is also still in full development at six years (Cekaite, 2013), so that the results here are not surprising.

The data analysed here are taken from conversations in NGT. They suggest that, in terms of the hypotheses proposed by Stivers et al. (2009), NGT is a language which allows overlap and shared floor. We know of spoken languages that do not show so much overlap in conversations, such as Swedish, but this has not yet been shown for a sign language. However, from personal observations and anecdotes we surmise that sign languages also seem to differ in the speed of adult-adult turn taking: ASL seems to be quicker for turn-taking than BSL for example. In general there seems to be support for their second hypothesis, that there is considerable cultural variability between languages. It is not yet known from documented research to what extent there are also cultural differences between individual sign languages in turn-taking or whether there are possible modality differences between spoken and signed languages.

Acknowledgment

We wish to express our thanks to students of Hogeschool Utrecht, University of Applied Sciences who assisted with transcription: Wieteke van Genderen, Yolanda Kriek, Marleen Steeloper, Andrea Heimenberg-Tholen and to Matthijs Terpstra, member of the Dutch Deaf community.

References

Bacchini, S, Kuiken, F., & Schoonen, R. (1995) Generalizability of spontaneous data: The effect of occasion and place on the speech production of children. *First Language* 15, 131–150. https://doi.org/10.1177/014272379501504401

Baker, A. E., & Van den Bogaerde, B. (2008). Codemixing in sign and words in input to and output from children. In C. Plaza Pust & E. Morales Lopez (Eds.), *Sign bilingualism: Language development, interaction and maintenance in language contact situations* (pp. 1–27). Amsterdam: John Benjamins. https://doi.org/10.1075/sibil.38.04bak

Baker, A. E. & Van den Bogaerde, B. (2012). Communicative interaction. In R. Pfau, M. Steinbach, & B. Woll (Eds.), *A handbook of sign linguistics* (pp. 489–512). Berlin: Mouton de Gruyter.

Baker, A., Van den Bogaerde, B., & Woll, B. (2009). Methods and procedures in sign language acquisition studies. In A. Baker & B. Woll (Eds.), *Sign language acquisition* (pp. 1–49). Amsterdam: John Benjamins. https://doi.org/10.1075/bct.14.03bak

Baker, C. (1977). Regulators and turn-taking in American Sign Language discourse. In L. A. Friedman (Ed.), *On the other hand* (pp. 2018–2236). New York, NY: Academic Press.

Barton, M. E., & Tomasello, M. (1991). Joint attention and conversation in Mother–Infant–Sibling Triads. *Child Development* 62(3), 517–529. https://doi.org/10.2307/1131127

Blain-Brière, B., Bouchard, C., & Bigras, N. (2014). The role of executive functions in the pragmatic skills of children aged 4–5. *Frontiers in Psychology* 5, 240. https://doi.org/10.3389/fpsyg.2014.00240.

Casillas, M. (2014). Turn-taking. In D. Matthews (Ed.) *Pragmatic development in first language acquisition* (pp. 53–70). Amsterdam: John Benjamins.

Casillas, M., Bobb, S. C. & Clark, E. V. (2016). Turn-taking, timing and planning in early language acquisition. *Journal of Child Language* 43, 1310–1337. https://doi.org/10.1017/S0305000915000689.

Cekaite, A. (2013). Child pragmatic development. In C. A. Chapelle (Ed.), *The encyclopedia of applied linguistics* (pp. 1–7). Malden, MA: Blackwell.
doi: https://doi.org/10.1002/9781405198431.wbeal0127

Coates, J. & Sutton-Spence, R. (2001). Turn-taking patterns in deaf conversation. *Journal of Sociolinguistics* 5(4), 507–529. https://doi.org/10.1111/1467-9481.00162

Cramér-Wolrath, E. (2011). Attention interchange at story-time: A case study from a deaf and hearing twin pair acquiring Swedish Sign Language in their deaf family. *Journal of Deaf Studies and Deaf Education* 17(2), 141–162. https://doi.org/10.1093/deafed/enr029

De Vos, C., Torreira, F., & Levinson, S. C. (2015). Turn-timing in signed conversations: Coordinating stroke-to-stroke boundaries. *Frontiers in Psychology* 6, 268. https://doi.org/10.3389/fpsyg.2015.00268

ELAN. <https://tla.mpi.nl/tools/tla-tools/elan/>

Filipi, A. (2014). Conversation analysis and pragmatic development. In D. Matthews (Ed.), *Pragmatic development in first language acquisition* (pp. 71–86). Amsterdam: John Benjamins.

Galloway, C., & Richards, B. J. (1994). *Input and interaction in language acquisition*. Cambridge: Cambridge University Press. https://doi.org/10.1017/CBO9780511620690

Garrod, S. & Pickering, M. J. (2009). Joint action, interactive alignment, and dialog. *Topics in Cognitive Science* 1, 292–304. https://doi.org/10.1111/j.1756-8765.2009.01020.x

Harris, M., Clibbens, J, Chasin, J. & Tibbitts, R. (1989). The social context of early sign language development. *First Language* 9(25), 81–97. https://doi.org/10.1177/014272378900902507

Hoza, J. (2007). *It is not what you sign, but how you sign it. Politeness in American Sign Language*. Washington, DC: Gallaudet University Press.

Kimmelman, V., & Pfau, R. (2016). Information structure in signed languages. In C. Féry & S. Ishihara (Eds.), *The Oxford handbook of information structure* (pp. 814–833). New York, NY: Oxford University Press. https://doi.org/10.1093/oxfordhb/9780199642670.013.001

Kotowicz, J. Woll, B., Herman, R., Schromová, M., Kiela-Turska, M. & Łacheta, J. (2017). Executive function in deaf native signing children: The relationship of language experience and cognition. Presentation at Formal and Experimental Advances in Sign Language Theory, June 2017.

Levinson, S. C., & Torreira, F. (2015). Timing in turn-taking and its implications for processing models of language. *Frontiers in Psychology* 6, 731. https://doi.org/10.3389/fpsyg.2015.00731

McCleary, L. E., & Leite, T. (2012). Turn-taking in Brazilian Sign Language: Evidence from overlap. *Journal of Interactional Research in Communication Disorders* 4(1), 124–153. https://doi.org/10.1558/jircd.v4i1.123

Peters, K. (n.d.). Hierarchy of social/pragmatic skills as related to the development of executive function. Retrieved at <https://www.seattlechildrens.org> (accessed February 2018).

Prinz, P. M. & Prinz, E. A. (1985). If only you could hear what I see. Discourse development in sign language. *Discourse Processes* 8, 1–19. https://doi.org/10.1080/01638538509544605

Rendle-Short, J., Skelt, L., & Bramley, N. (2015). Speaking to twin children: Evidence against the "Impoverishment" thesis. *Research on Language and Interaction* 48(1), 79–99. https://doi.org/10.1080/08351813.2015.993846

Roos, C., Cramér-Wolrath, E., & Falkman, K. W. (2016). Intersubjective interaction between deaf parents/deaf infants during the infants' first 18 months. *Journal of Deaf Studies and Deaf Education* 21(1), 11–22. <https://academic.oup.com/jdsde/article/21/1/11/2404191> https://doi.org/10.1093/deafed/env034

Schegloff, E. A. (2000). Overlapping talk and the organization of turn-taking for conversation. *Language in Society* 29(1), 1–63. https://doi.org/10.1017/S0047404500001019

Schick, B., De Villiers, P., De Villiers, J., & Hoffmeister, R. (2007). Language and Theory of Mind: A study of deaf children. *Child Development* 78(2), 376–396. https://doi.org/10.1111/j.1467-8624.2007.01004.x

Stivers, Y., Enfield, N. J., Brown, P., Englert, C., Hayashi, M., Heinemann, T., Hoymann, G., Rossano, F., De Ruiter, J.-P., Yoon, K. R., & Levinson, S. (2009). Universals and cultural variation in turn taking in conversation. *PNAS* 106(26), 10587–10592. <http://www.pnas.org/content/106/26/10587.full.pdf> https://doi.org/10.1073/pnas.0903616106

Sutton Spence, R., & Woll, B. (1999). *The linguistics of British Sign Language: An introduction.* Cambridge: Cambridge University Press. https://doi.org/10.1017/CBO9781139167048

Tomasello, T., Manle, S., & Kruger, A. (1986). Linguistic environment of 1- to 2-year-old twins. *Developmental Psychology* 22(2), 169–176. https://doi.org/10.1037/0012-1649.22.2.169

Van den Bogaerde, B. (2000) *Input and interaction in deaf families* (PhD dissertation). University of Amsterdam. <wwwlot.let.uu.nl> https://doi.org/10.1075/sll.3.1.12bog

Van den Bogaerde, B. & Baker, A. E. (2002). Are young deaf children bilingual? In G. Morgan & B. Woll (Eds.), *Directions in sign language acquisition* (pp. 183–206). Amsterdam: John Benjamins. https://doi.org/10.1075/tilar.2.11bog

Van den Bogaerde, B. & Baker, A. E. (2006). Code mixing in mother–child interaction in deaf families. *Sign Language and Linguistics* 8(1/2), 155–178.

Van den Bogaerde, B. & Baker, A. E. (2014). Eye-gaze in turn taking in sign language interaction. Paper to IASCL, July 2014, Amsterdam.

Van Herreweghe, M. (2002). Turn-taking mechanisms and active participation in meetings with Deaf and hearing participants in Flanders. In C. Lucas (Ed.), *Turn-taking, fingerspelling, and contact in signed languages: Sociolinguistics in Deaf communities* (pp. 73–103). Washington, DC: Gallaudet University Press.

Wilbur, R., & Petitto, L. A. (1983/2009). Discourse structure in American Sign Language conversations (or, how to know a conversation when you see one). *Discourse Processes* 6(3), 225–2241. Retrieved at <http://www.tandfonline.com/doi/abs/10.1080/01638538309544565> (accessed August 2017). https://doi.org/10.1080/01638538309544565

Woll, B. (1978). Structure and function in language acquisition. In *The development of communication* (pp. 321–331). New York, NY: Wiley.

Woolfe, T., Want, S. C., & Siegal, M. (2003). Siblings and Theory of Mind in deaf native children. *Journal of Deaf Studies and Deaf Education* 8(3), 340–347. https://doi.org/10.1093/deafed/eng023

CHAPTER 4

The assessment of signed languages

Ros Herman, Nicola Grove, Tobias Haug, Wolfgang Mann
and Philip Prinz

Despite the large number of assessments available to measure spoken language
acquisition, until relatively recently no assessments were available that could
be used to evaluate deaf children's sign language acquisition. This is despite
the fact that sign language has been used with deaf children in educational
contexts for many years, and that deaf children are widely acknowledged to
be at risk for language development. However, development of sign language
assessments presents unique methodological challenges, due to factors such as
our relatively limited knowledge of language acquisition in sign, and also to the
nature and size of the Deaf community – the latter presenting specific challenges
when standardising measures. This chapter will present two current areas of
research related to sign language assessment, drawing on expertise from the
UK, USA and Germany.

Introduction

An important element in the study of deaf children's language is the possibility of
assessing level of development and monitoring change. Despite the large number
of assessments available to measure spoken language acquisition, until relatively
recently no published assessments were available for practitioners to evaluate
deaf children's sign language acquisition. This was even though signed languages
have been used with deaf children in educational contexts for many years, and
deaf children are widely acknowledged to be at risk for language development
(Herman, 2015; see Chapter 2 by Harris & Clibbens and Chapter 7 by Morgan,
Jones & Botting, this volume). The development of sign language assessments
presents unique methodological challenges to test developers, in part because
of the relatively limited research base on language acquisition in different sign
languages, and also the size and nature of the Deaf community (Woolfe, Herman,
Roy, & Woll, 2010).

https://doi.org/10.1075/tilar.25.04her

Bencie Woll has been a motivating force in this area from the outset. As co-author of the first standardised assessments of sign language acquisition (Herman, Holmes, & Woll, 1999; Herman et al., 2004), this work has stimulated colleagues to address the topic in different sign languages around the world (see Enns et al., 2016 for a recent overview). Drawing on expertise from the UK, USA and Switzerland, this chapter reviews recent developments in sign language assessment. These include methodological issues encountered when designing and using the new generation of web-based sign language tests, developments in the dynamic assessment of sign language, and the application of assessments to diverse groups of sign language users, encompassing deaf and hearing children, adults with intellectual disabilities who use sign, and hearing adults learning sign as a second language.

The first published assessments of sign language acquisition

By the 1990s, sign bilingual education was increasingly used with deaf children in the UK and elsewhere, with a main objective to develop first language skills in sign as a basis for subsequent acquisition of a second spoken and/or written language (Johnson et al., 1989; Kyle, 1987; Pickersgill & Gregory, 1998 and Tang et al. Chapter 10, this volume). At that time, there were no tests of sign language acquisition for practitioners to use to ascertain whether one of the key aims of the sign educational approach was achievable, although some tests had been developed and used for research purposes. In the absence of available tests, deaf children's language was assessed in a variety of informal ways. A survey of UK schools by Herman (1998a) identified inconsistent approaches to sign language assessment. In some, a lack of practitioner confidence and skills meant that the whole area of sign language assessment was overlooked, with practitioners focusing exclusively on deaf children's skills in other language domains, i.e. spoken and written English. In other schools, staff had translated tests of spoken language, or identified specific features of sign language that differed from school to school, and were evaluating them in unsystematic and unreliable ways, rendering comparison between children across different schools impossible (ibid.)

These early insights paved the way for the development of the first two standardized tests of any sign language: the British Sign Language Receptive Skills Test (BSL RST, Herman et al., 1999) and the BSL Production Test (BSL PT, Herman et al., 2004). Both tests were initially developed on native signers and subsequently used with a broader sample including deaf children from hearing families to develop norms (Herman & Woll, 1998). Although the final standardization samples in each test were small in comparison with tests of spoken languages, which typically include hundreds of children, they represented significant proportions of the deaf signing population in the UK. These tests offered a first opportunity for practitioners to evaluate deaf children's sign language acquisition in comparison to deaf norms, and by default, to evaluate whether sign bilingual education could successfully achieve good levels of sign language in all deaf children.

A key question in the development of the BSL RST was how to deliver the test in a uniform way. Spoken language measures maintain a standardized approach to test administration by testers reading written instructions to children. Sign languages have no written form, and preliminary pilot work with the BSL RST identified inconsistencies in test administration as a result (Herman, 1998b). By filming test items and presenting them to children on video, this first challenge was overcome and brought with it other benefits. The use of a video-based assessment minimized the need for tester skill. As a result, the test became popular and was widely used throughout the UK, and has since been adapted to other sign languages (e.g. American Sign Language, ASL: Enns & Herman, 2011; Australian Sign Language, Auslan: Johnston, 2004; German Sign Language, *Deutsche Gebärdensprache*, DGS: Haug, 2011; Japanese Sign Language: Wataru 2012, 2016; Polish Sign Language, *Polski Język Migowy*, PJM: Kotowicz, Schromova, Herman & Woll, submitted; Spanish Sign Language, *Lengua de Signas Espanola*, LSE: Valmaseda, Perez, Ramírez & Montero, 2013).

In contrast to the BSL RST, for the BSL PT, practitioners must be trained in its use. This is because tester skill is essential when evaluating expressive sign language skills. The training course continues to recruit deaf and hearing staff from different professional backgrounds (e.g. teachers, speech and language therapists, deaf instructors) and provides attendees with knowledge that is essential not only to using the test, but also to their roles as assessors of sign language acquisition, thereby addressing some of the concerns about conducting assessments of sign language raised by practitioners (Herman, 1998a). Course participants receive training in sign linguistics, sign language acquisition, narrative skills and their development, and principles of testing. Attendees are assessed on their ability to administer the test, analyse narrative samples reliably, and report accurately on findings before becoming registered test users. Recent developments include a follow-on course in designing and delivering language therapy in BSL for children identified with language deficits (Hoskin, 2017).

The BSL RST has recently been redeveloped for delivery via a web-based assessment portal (see Figure 1; Herman, Rowley & Woll, 2015), which has brought with it a new means of collecting normative data.

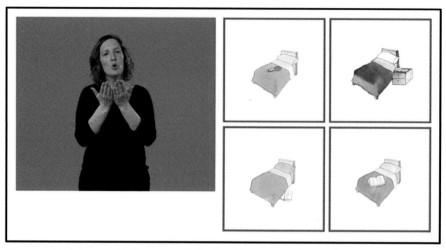

Figure 1. Web-based BSL Receptive Skills Test (Herman et al., 2015)

Comparing children's assessment scores before and after a period of significant change in the field of childhood deafness (see Chapters 1 and 2 by Harris & Clibbens), which has included the introduction of newborn hearing screening and earlier use of better amplification devices, provides insights into the population of sign language users with whom the test is currently used (Herman & Curtin, 2017). We now turn to other advances in web-based sign language assessment across different countries.

Methodological issues in web-based sign language assessment for deaf students

Technologies have revolutionized the education of deaf students (Keating & Mirus, 2004; Stinson, 2010) and transformed the process of assessment for hearing and deaf students in a range of academic-related domains (e.g., achievement, college entrance exams, aptitude, reading), including language. In comparison with traditional non-computer-based forms of evaluation, the emergence of computer and web-based/online testing offers advantages and challenges for students, teachers, and educational/clinical specialists.

Haug (2015) conducted an international online survey of sign language test developers and reported findings from nineteen research groups from ten different countries (Australia, Canada, Czech Republic, Ethiopia, Germany, France, Iceland, Netherlands, United Kingdom, and USA). Overall, respondents reported advantages of using computer- or web-based formats, including automatic scoring and analysis of test results, ease of data collection and test delivery, accessibility of tests in varied locations, and a standardized test format that improved reliability and validity. In terms of challenges, survey participants mentioned difficulties with the technical infrastructure (i.e., dated hardware and software, server connection problems), security/data protection issues, limited financial resources for employing programmers, the design of the web-based test interface, and the quality of recorded videos (potentially affected the accuracy of assessment). Overall, many negative issues regarding assessment of students' language abilities (spoken, written, and signed) have been greatly improved and enhanced by internet technology, and as a consequence, web-based assessments are widely used in the field of second language learning (Chapelle & Douglas, 2006; Chapelle & Voss, 2016) and increasingly with hearing children with suspected language impairments (Waite, Theodoros, Russell, & Cahill, 2010).

To illustrate some of the most relevant issues in sign language testing, we present two examples: the web-based BSL Vocabulary Test, (BSL-VT, Mann, 2009) and the Software-based Assessment of ASL Abilities (SAASLA LLC, 2015). The web-based BSL-VT was designed to assess deaf children's vocabulary knowledge in BSL "by specifically measuring the degree of strength of the mappings between form and meaning for items in the core lexicon" (Mann & Marshall, 2012, p. 1031). Mann utilized an online format to investigate mapping between phonological form and meaning of signs in BSL, both receptively and expressively. Students use computers (Mac or PC) connected to the internet and are asked to select either an image corresponding to a stimulus sign or a sign corresponding to a stimulus image (see Figure 2). During the receptive task, student responses are automatically saved onto an Excel datasheet on the web server. For the production tasks, children produce a sign corresponding to the stimulus image and responses are

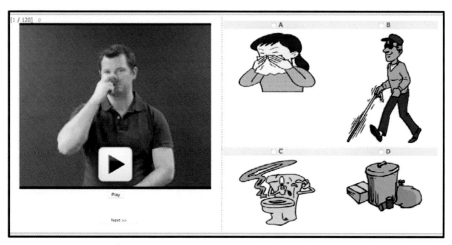

Figure 2. BSL Vocabulary Test (Mann, 2009)

entered manually with English glosses by the researcher during test administration and automatically saved to the database on the web server. The *BSL-VT* has been adapted and translated into ASL (Mann, Roy, & Morgan, 2016).

The SAASLA is a norm-referenced online assessment of ASL that can be used by teachers and educational specialists to assess a deaf student's sign language abilities. The test consists of multiple-choice items assessing ASL abilities, including both manual and non-manual elements across three overlapping linguistic domains: (1) the phonological structure of signs and the lexicon; (2) morphology and syntax, and (3) semantics/pragmatics/discourse (for a linguistic description of sign language grammar, see Chapter 6 Lillo-Martin et al., this volume). Test items are derived from established linguistic categories that characterize all languages and which are supported by ASL linguistic, pedagogical, and developmental psycholinguistic research.

As with any online project, establishing a reliable and workable feature set is important. An online language test requires some technological features that other online services do not need. For example, a scheduler for online assessments can be useful for setting up assessment appointments so that a tester can plan which students will be taking the assessment and when. This may be important where a school has a limited number of computers with adequate quality video monitors, or where there are concerns about the network bandwidth and therefore the number of simultaneous assessment sessions must be restricted.

The biggest challenge in creating any sign language assessment tool is the design of test items and validating the instrument for reliability and validity. Important issues include identifying specific linguistic categories and maintaining an even distribution of items for each; establishing order of difficulty across test items; utilizing native signers to develop and present test items; employing different types of stimuli for assessment items (i.e. signed, static pictures, animation); and considering cultural variations of signs. In summary, the arrival of web-based language assessment tools opens a new chapter in sign language assessment.

Dynamic assessment

In addition to different test formats, assessment of language development has begun to incorporate methods based more on the potential of a child to learn rather than their current level. This is because many hearing children with culturally and linguistically diverse backgrounds perform poorly on standardized tests of English, either due to a lack of familiarity with standardized testing (Peña, Iglesias, & Lidz, 2001) or differences between children's language experiences at home and in school (Hart, 1995; Flanagan, Ortiz, & Alfonso, 2013; Schieffelin & Ochs, 1986).

As a result, many bilingual hearing children end up being misdiagnosed with a language impairment. Deaf children whose first language is a signed language are similarly challenging to assess, especially when using standardized tests designed to measure spoken language.

While more tests of sign language acquisition have been developed in recent years, there are limitations to the type of tests available, and an interest in alternative approaches to assessment has increased. Rather than measuring learning outcomes at a particular point in time, alternative approaches have focused on assessing the learning process. One such approach is dynamic assessment. Dynamic assessment combines teaching and assessment within a single procedure to measure learning potential and evaluate the enhanced performance that results from assisted learning. The most common formats of dynamic assessment include test-teach-retest and gradual prompting (Hasson, 2017). During test-teach-retest, the child is asked to carry out a task and receives prompts where necessary. The child is then retested on the same/comparable task and progress is monitored along with the level of prompting required. During graduated prompting, there is no pre-test. Instead, the child is given a task and receives prompts as needed, arranged in a hierarchy from least to most supportive to achieve success. The number of prompts required to enable the child to succeed is recorded.

Dynamic assessment draws conceptually on Vygotsky's zone of proximal development (Vygotsky, 1978), which proposes that a child can develop higher mental functioning through collaboration/interaction with a more experienced peer or adult. Others (Feuerstein, 1979; Lidz, 1987, 1991) have adapted this concept to describe the interaction during mediation (Mediated Learning Experience, MLE), which is part of the teaching phase of dynamic interaction (Hasson & Joffe, 2007; Peña et al., 2006; Peña, Gillam, & Bedore, (2014). Here, mediator and child engage in learning experiences that aim to teach the child problem-solving strategies and/or principles of task solution, both of which are key to successful test-taking performance. For example, in a mediation session targeting semantic categories, a task to introduce the child to this concept may involve sorting objects based on their size, shape or colour. The mediator, who is also the assessor, monitors any changes in the child's learning strategies and/or signs of increased competence in response to MLE which leads to an evaluation of the child's learning ability, along with their potential to benefit from instruction (Feuerstein, 1979; Haywood & Wingenfeld, 1992; Lidz, 1987, 1991).

Although the number of studies is at this point quite limited and based on child participants who use a variety of communication approaches, there are two principal strands of research examining deaf children's response to dynamic assessment. One strand has explored dynamic assessment of cognitive skills in deaf children. Here, studies have mainly compared dynamic and static assessments of deaf children's learning potential, with a particular focus on performance on (verbal) IQ tests as a measure of cognitive functioning, on which deaf children typically perform poorly (see Chapter 7 Morgan; Hubert & Koeler, 1984; Katz & Buchholz, 1984; Lidz, 2004; Olswang & Bain, 1996; Tzuriel & Caspri, 1992).

The second strand of research focuses on the use of dynamic assessment within a language-learning context (signed or spoken). Here, most studies have applied a test-teach-retest paradigm to examine children's responsiveness to mediation and the level of effort required by the mediator (Asad, Hand, Fairgray, & Purdy, 2013; Mann, Peña, & Morgan, 2014; 2015). For example, Mann et al. (2014, 2015) used scripted MLE sessions to target lexical-semantic organization, first in a small pilot with two children (Mann, Peña, & Morgan, 2014) and then with a larger group of children (N = 37) with varying language ability (Mann, Peña, & Morgan, 2015). In both studies, two sessions were delivered in ASL by one (Mann et al., 2014) or two mediators (Mann et al., 2015). The mediators were fluent ASL users (children of deaf adults – CODAs).

Activities in the MLE sessions included sorting objects, pictures and ASL signs into semantic categories. At the end of each session, mediators used the Modifiability Observation Form (MOF, Peña & Villarreal, 2000), a checklist targeting child behavioural and cognitive features, to rate children's responses to mediation (i.e., child modifiability). Children's language skills were measured by performance on an ASL proficiency rating scale, developed as part of these studies, and recommendations/concerns by the speech-language therapist and teacher. Results showed that modifiability ratings were highly sensitive to language ability. Furthermore, significant group differences emerged between strong and weak language users on both behavioral (e.g., anxiety, motivation) and cognitive (e.g., problem-solving, verbal mediation) measures of the MOF. These findings are in line with studies that have used dynamic assessment in language-learning contexts with hearing children (e.g., Kapantzoglou, Restrepo, & Thompson, 2012; Peña, Reséndiz, & Gillam, 2007; Ukrainetz et al., 2000).

One advantage of dynamic assessment is that it enables mediators, who are blind to a child's (dis)ability, to accurately judge which children require more support and those who are less responsive to any support provided (Mann et al., 2014). Moreover, as demonstrated by Azad et al. (2013) and Mann et al. (2014, 2015), the use of dynamic assessment is not limited to hearing populations or spoken language but can be extended to deaf children including those who use sign, and its use tailored to an individual child's language preference.

While there are advantages of dynamic assessment over static tests, dynamic assessment works best when used in combination with existing norm-referenced and descriptive testing practices. This combined approach enables practitioners in schools to pinpoint specific difficulties a pupil may encounter when trying out a new task and draw more valid conclusions regarding the language-learning ability of such learners. However, a remaining challenge is to develop and maintain strong(er) links between assessment and intervention. To practitioners and/or parents, there may not always be a clear connection between the results of a test and classroom practice, in particular if the amount of information provided and the jargon used make it difficult to understand (Deutsch & Reynolds, 2000). While more research is needed on how to implement dynamic assessment in the classroom in a meaningful way, there are some available materials, e.g., a checklist of cognitive learning principles, to help the assessor record information and provide feedback about good starting points, e.g., Lauchlan & Carrigan (2013); Hasson (2017). For a more detailed discussion, see Mann (2018).Two further areas where sign language assessment has provided useful insights are signers who have intellectual disabilities and hearing adult sign language learners.

Assessment of signers who have intellectual disabilities

People with intellectual disabilities[1] who sign are a varied population and constitute approximately 6–7% of the deaf population (Bunch & Melnyk, 1989). They include those who are born deaf or develop deafness later in life, as well as others who have hearing that is adequate to process speech yet use manual signs to support their understanding or expressive language. Traditionally, this latter group are classed as users of augmentative and alternative communication (AAC) and their signing is developed through forms of sign supported speech (where spoken English is used, known as Sign Supported English, SSE), and usually using a key word system such as Makaton (see Meuris et al., 2015; Grove & Walker, 1990).

Hearing and deaf children and adults with intellectual disabilities tend to have high levels of language and communication difficulties, whether in sign or speech (Emerson, 2007), exacerbated by low expectations (e.g. Campbell et al., 2003); learned passivity (e.g. Basil, 1992); and an overemphasis on very basic communication functions such as requests, particularly for those with severe difficulties (e.g. Carbone et al., 2010). Some have intrinsic problems, such as poor oral motor and fine motor co-ordination, resulting in poor intelligibility of speech or sign; complications caused by specific neurodevelopmental difficulties, or generalised brain damage.

---

1. An intellectual disability is defined as reduced cognitive ability and difficulty with everyday activities which affects someone for their whole life. A social perspective emphasises that disability results from the interactions between an individual with impairments and the environment in which they function.

There are certain principles of assessment of language and cognition that apply regardless of the level of intellectual functioning or deafness. As with dynamic assessment, assessment should be about potential for achievement, not simply deficit focused. With deaf individuals in signing environments, existing standardised sign language assessments can be used (Enns et al., 2013; Herman et al., 1999, 2004; Woolfe et al., 2010), although norms based on typically developing individuals should be used with caution. Test results should always be supplemented with information about functional knowledge and use of signs. This may be obtained by observation, backed up by reports from families and staff, which provides insights not only into what the person with intellectual disability is doing, but the nature of the input by interactive partners, and the quality of the signing environment (e.g. number of people who sign, level of fluency in sign), all of which are crucial. If the input is poor and the culture is overwhelmingly biased towards spoken language, there will be little motivation for people to use the signs they know (Rombouts, Maes, & Zink, 2017; Woll & Barnett, 1998).

Gesture and speech form an integrated system (McNeill, 1992), and for the majority of the population of hearing signers with intellectual disabilities, many of whom struggle to communicate using solely spoken language, it is therefore important to consider how the two systems interact. It is essential to take account of modality use and modality dependence in different communication situations. For language comprehension, it may sometimes be appropriate to look at the individual's use of sign language, signed supported speech, and speech alone, particularly to ascertain the optimal input. For expressive communication, both sign and speech output should be recorded and analysed, and it is helpful to be familiar with basic multimodal transcription conventions (see von Tetzchner & Basil, 2011).

Hearing and deaf signers with intellectual disabilities often have impaired motor skills, due either to problems of dyspraxia and low muscle tone, which affect the parameters of sign production: handshape (whole handshapes being easier to form than those involving complex finger isolations), movement (simple directional movements being easier than alternating movements, for example), location (easier for locations within the visual field than out), and orientation (reverse orientation being particularly difficult). Because these four parameters interact, there is considerable redundancy available, which means that it is possible to recognise the meaning of a sign even when one or more are incorrectly produced (more so than for spoken language). For such individuals, it is useful to consult with a physiotherapist and occupational therapist as part of the assessment process and look at what the individual can do in imitation (whole sign and handshape independently) and how they use their hands in functional everyday activities as well as in spontaneous communication (Grove, Darke, Brownlie, & Bloomberg, in press).

Research into child language acquisition shows that mastery of a large vocabulary is one of the keys to the development of semantic networks, phonology and grammar (see inter alia Marchman & Fernald, 2008; Morgan et al., 2015). The sign vocabularies of hearing signers with intellectual disability are often small, so account should be taken of what they know, what they understand, how vocabulary is distributed across modalities, and how they use what they know. A sign-adapted test such as the BSL version of the MacArthur Communicative Development Inventories (Woolfe et al., 2010) may be useful. Alternatively, a customised vocabulary checklist can be used for staff and families to fill in, with columns for sign and speech. For those with vocabularies smaller than 50 items, staff and families can be asked to list signs and words in daily use. These should be supplemented with informal testing using a checklist supported by pictures or photos because other signs, e.g. those learned at school, may be remembered even though they are not used in the current setting.

Relatively few people with intellectual disability in sign supported speech programmes and oral environments progress from single words to sign combinations or sentences (Kiernan et al., 1982; Grove & Dockrell, 2000; Grove & Woll, 2017). Many will combine sign and speech, or even sign one part and say another, so again it is important to ensure that both modalities are recorded. For those unable to be tested with standardised measures, an informal assessment approach that provides a dynamic context may be successful, for example, use of barrier communication games; describing a picture that the tester has to draw, or describing animated activity (computer games or films). Rudd, Grove and Pring (2007) described a procedure for testing and eliciting sign combinations using objects and actions contrastively (e.g. make the PLANE/BALL + FLY/BOUNCE). Although not all people with intellectual disabilities produce signed sentences, testers with in depth knowledge of sign linguistics may spot creative modifications to signs that are effective in extending the range of meanings expressed.

The ability to produce a narrative to tell another person about an experience is arguably one of the most important communication skills to develop, associated with emotional well-being, forming relationships, identity and self-esteem and self-advocacy (Grove, 2012; Ochs & Capps, 2001; Stefánsdóttir & Traustadóttir, 2015). Picture-book based assessments involving retelling or story generation, such as the Frog Story (Mercer Mayer, 1969), which has been widely used with hearing and deaf children, are less suited to this population for a variety of reasons. For example, narratives are more complete when told to a naive listener who clearly does not know or see the original, and where the stimulus materials are dynamic and interesting enough to warrant the effort of telling (see Grove & Woll, 2017 for discussion). The film-based task in the BSL PT (Herman et al., 2004) was originally developed to assess narrative skills in signing children with intellectual disabilities and has been successfully used in this context (Grove, 1995).

Importantly, investigations of signing in individuals with intellectual disabilities can be revealing about the nature of language and language disabilities. A study of hearing twins with Down syndrome who communicated with their Deaf parents in sign language led to insights into underlying and cross-modal linguistic problems in children with Down syndrome, whose deficits had hitherto been considered specific to auditory processing (Woll & Grove, 1996). Subsequent investigations with individuals who have diverse needs and abilities, many inspired by Bencie have made further contributions.

Assessment of adult learners of a sign language

Compared to the assessment of deaf signing children, the assessment of adult learners of a sign language as a second or foreign language is a relatively new topic within sign language test research. With the increasing awareness and implementation of the Common European Framework of Reference (CEFR; Council of Europe, 2009) in sign language teaching (e.g. in sign language interpreter training), testing of adult learners has become more visible as a topic in recent years through projects such as ProSign 1 and ProSign 2 <http://www.ecml.at/pro-sign>.

There are two distinct groups of adult learners of sign languages. One comprises deaf people who have acquired a sign language as a first language (L1) and who are learning a second sign language as adults, i.e. where the second sign language is in the same modality (M1) as the L1. The second group comprises hearing individuals who have acquired a spoken language as an L1 and who learn a sign language later in life, i.e. the sign language is acquired in a different, second modality (M2) (Emmorey, Borinstein, Thompson, & Gollan, 2008).

Very little research has been carried out on sign language tests for adult learners. One of the few examples is the Sign Language Proficiency Interview (SLPI; Newell, Caccamise, Boardman, & Holcomb, 1983). The SLPI makes use of an interview format, which is video-recorded for later analysis. The SLPI has been adapted to other sign languages, such as Sign Language of the Netherlands (*Nederlandse Gebarentaal*, NGT; Van den Broek-Laven, Boers-Visker, & Van den Bogaerde, 2014) and is currently also being adapted to Swiss German Sign Language (*Deutschschweizerische Gebärdensprache*, DSGS). Other examples of sign language tests targeting adult learners are the Sentence Reproduction Test for ASL (Hauser, Supalla, & Bavellier, 2008), designed as a "global, objective assessment ASL proficiency test" (p. 171) and the ASL Discrimination Test (Bochner et al., 2016), which tests "learners' ability to discriminate phonological and morphophonological contrasts in ASL, [and] provides an objective overall measure of ASL proficiency" (p. 473). While the Sentence Reproduction Test is a more research-oriented assessment, the ASL Discrimination Test is intended to be a more functional assessment of the ASL proficiency of adult deaf learners.

Sign language test developers face methodological challenges when they develop sign language tests, independent of whether the target group is children or adults (Haug & Mann, 2008). These may arise due to limitations in research on sign languages in general, or because no corpus or reference grammar is available. A corpus can be used to generate sign frequency lists which in turn can inform the development of a vocabulary test. For example, there exist corpora for BSL (Fenlon, Schembri, Rentelis, Vinson, & Cormier, 2014) and DGS (Hanke, 2017) which can be used as a resource to inform test development. Another example is from the Netherlands where the University of Applied Sciences in Utrecht trains teachers and interpreters in NGT in a four-year bachelor's program. As part of the process of aligning their curriculum to the CEFR, the university needed to develop CEFR-level-appropriate tests (Van den Broek-Laven et al., 2014). Apart from productive measures, the university was interested in developing NGT comprehension tests for the different CEFR levels. Due to the lack of research on different text types in signed languages, they applied a set of different linguistic criteria that were identified during a literature review which served as indicators for signed text difficulty (Van den Broek-Laven et al., 2014):

1. Sign familiarity
2. Morpheme-sign rate: "the average number of morphemes per sign over a minute of text" (Van den Broek-Laven et al., 2014, p. 69)
3. Use of space, e.g., to establish a referent; use of verbs.
4. Non-manual components, e.g., to mark a question; to express negation.

The signed texts that were used in the different levels of NGT training served as basis for testing these criteria. As a result of testing these criteria, the best predictors of text difficulty were sign familiarity and morpheme-sign rate. As for use of space, the use of agreement verbs, spatial verbs, non-manual markers, and the use of anaphoric reference were good indicators of text difficulty and increased over the different CEFR levels A1-B2 in the course of the BA training at Utrecht University of Applied Sciences.

Overall conclusions

The field of sign language assessment is young. As more tests are developed and older tests are updated, the possibilities of newer technologies are increasingly exploited. Paradoxically, as the numbers of sign language assessments grow, earlier diagnosis of deafness and improvements in amplification technology in many parts of the world now mean that fewer deaf children use sign language than previously. Amongst the challenges this presents is how to update test norms on a diminishing population of sign language users. The increased use of web-based tests offers a potential solution to this.

The scope of sign language assessment is now being extended to different groups of sign language users. Although available measures focus exclusively on sign language, not all children who use sign are users of the full language. Many deaf children and hearing children with and without intellectual disabilities use SSE. Future assessments need to consider how to address the full communicative repertoire of those who combine sign and speech. With reference to the measurement of L2 learners of sign languages, clearer definitions of the components of sign language proficiency are needed, framed within a model of communicative language ability (e.g., Bachman, 1996; Canale & Swain, 1980), as for spoken languages. Moreover, future research in this field should go beyond methodological issues and also take account of learners' feedback and perspectives to improve the validity of sign language tests.

Measures of sign language are clearly important to child and adult signers, their families and the professionals who work with them, but also bring value to research. Recent research with child populations has used available assessments to differentiate delays in sign language acquisition, typically found in many deaf children in hearing families, from more specific difficulties with language learning (Herman et al., 2014; Herman, Rowley, Mason, & Morgan, 2014 and see Chapter 5 by Marshall et al., this volume). Research in the emerging field of sign language acquisition in adult learners may in future lead to a better understanding of the process of bimodal language acquisition, and in turn influence the development of new measures.

References

Asad, A. N., Hand, L., Fairgray, L., & Purdy, S. C. (2013). The use of dynamic assessment to evaluate narrative language learning in children with hearing loss: Three case studies. *Child Language Teaching and Therapy* 29(3), 319–342. https://doi.org/10.1177/0265659012467994

Bachman, L. F., & Palmer, A. (1996). *Language testing in practice*. Oxford: Oxford University Press.

Basil, C. (1992). Social interaction and learned helplessness in severely disabled children. *Augmentative and Alternative Communication* 8, 188–199.
https://doi.org/10.1080/07434619212331276183

Bochner, J. H., Samar, V. J., Hauser, P. C., Garrison, W. M., Searls, J. M., & Sanders, C. A. (2016). Validity of the American Sign Language Discrimination Test. *Language Testing* 33(4), 473–495. https://doi.org/10.1177/0265532215590849

Bunch, G. O., & Melnyk, T. L. (1989). A review of the evidence for a learning-disabled, hearing impaired sub-group. *American Annals of the Deaf* 134, 297–300. https://doi.org/10.1353/aad.2012.0547

Campbell, J., Gilmore, L., & Cuskelly, M. (2003). Changing student teachers' attitudes towards disability and inclusion. *Journal of Intellectual and Developmental Disability* 28, 369–379. https://doi.org/10.1080/13668250310001616407

Canale, M., & Swain, M. (1980). Theoretical bases of communicative approaches to second language teaching and testing. *Applied Linguistics* 1,1–47. https://doi.org/10.1093/applin/1.1.1

Carbone, V., Sweeney-Kirwan, E., Attanasio, V., & Kasper, T. (2010). Increasing the vocal responses of children with autism and developmental disabilities using manual sign mand training and prompt delay. *Journal of Behavior Analysis* 43, 703–709.

Chapelle, C. A., & Douglas, D. (2006). *Assessing language through computer technology*. Cambridge: Cambridge University Press. https://doi.org/10.1017/CBO9780511733116

Chapelle, C. A., & Voss, E. (2016). 20 years of technology and language assessment in language learning & technology. *Language Learning & Technology* 20(2), 116–128.

Council of Europe (2009). *Common European framework of reference for languages: Learning, teaching, assessment*. Cambridge: Cambridge University Press.

Deutsch, R., & Reynolds, Y. (2000). The use of dynamic assessment by educational psychologists in the UK. *Educational Psychology in Practice* 16(3), 311–331. https://doi.org/10.1080/713666083

Emerson, E. (2007). Poverty and people with intellectual disabilities. *Mental Retardation and Developmental Disabilities Research Reviews*, 13, 107–113. doi: https://doi.org/10.1002/mrdd.20144

Emmorey, K., Borinstein, H. B., Thompson, R., & Gollan, T. H. (2008). Bimodal bilingualism. *Bilingualism: Language and Cognition* 11(1), 43–61. https://doi.org/10.1017/S1366728907003203

Enns, C., Haug, T., Herman, R., Hoffmeister, R. J., Mann, W., & Mcquarrie, L. (2016). Exploring signed language assessment tools in Europe and North America. In M. Marschark, V. Lampropoulou, & E. K. Skordilis (Eds.), *Diversity in deaf education* (pp. 171–218). New York, NY: Oxford University Press. https://doi.org/10.1093/acprof:oso/9780190493073.003.0007

Enns, C., & Herman, R. (2011). Adapting the assessing British Sign Language development: Receptive Skills Test into American Sign Language. *Journal of Deaf Studies and Deaf Education* 16(3), 362–374. https://doi.org/10.1093/deafed/enr004

Enns, C. E., Zimmer, K., Boudreault, P., Rabu, S., & Broszeit, C. (2013). *American Sign Language Receptive Skills Test*. Winnipeg, MB: Northern Signs Research.

Fenlon, J., Schembri, A., Rentelis, R., Vinson, D., & Cormier, K. (2014). Using conversational data to determine lexical frequency in British Sign Language: The influence of text type. *Lingua* 143, 187–202. https://doi.org/10.1016/j.lingua.2014.02.003

Feuerstein, R., Rand, Y., & Hoffman, M. B. (1979). *The dynamic assessment of retarded performers: The Learning Potential Assessment Device, theory, instruments, and techniques*. Baltimore, MD: University Park Press.

Flanagan, D. P., Ortiz, S. O., & Alfonso, V. C. (2013). *Essentials of cross-battery assessment*. Hoboken, NJ: John Wiley & Sons.

Grove, N. (1990) Developing intelligible signs with learning-disabled students: A review of the literature and an assessment procedure. *British Journal of Disorders of Communication* 25, 265–293. https://doi.org/10.3109/13682829009011978

Grove, N. (1995). *An analysis of the linguistic skills of signers with learning disabilities* (Unpublished PhD dissertation). London University.

Grove, N. (2012) Story, agency and meaning making: Narrative models and the social inclusion of people with severe and profound intellectual disabilities. *Journal of Religion, Disability and Health* 16, 334–351. https://doi.org/10.1080/15228967.2012.731887

Grove, N., Darke, L., Brownlie, E. & Bloomberg, K. (in press). Assessment and intervention for problems in sign production. In N. Grove & K. Launonen (Eds.), *Manual sign acquisition by children with developmental disabilities*. New York, NY: Nova Science Publishers.

Grove, N. & Dockrell, J. (2000) Multi-sign combinations by children with intellectual impairments: An analysis of language skills. *Journal of Language, Speech & Hearing Research* 43, 309–323. https://doi.org/10.1044/jslhr.4302.309

Grove, N. & Woll, B. (2017) Assessing language skills in adult key word signers with intellectual disabilities: Insights from sign linguistics. *Research in Developmental Disabilities* 62, 174–183. https://doi.org/10.1016/j.ridd.2017.01.017

Hanke, T. (2017). Wörterbuch ohne Wörter? Zum Entstehen eines Wörterbuches der Deutschen Gebärdensprache [A dictionary without words? On the creation of a dictionary for German Sign Language]. In Heidelberger Akademie der Wissenschaften (Ed.), *Jahrbuch der Heidelberger Akademie der Wissenschaften für 2016* (pp. 84–88). Heidelberg: Universitätsverlag Winter.

Hart, B., & Risley, T. R. (1995). *Meaningful differences in the everyday experience of young American children*. Baltimore, MD: Paul H. Brookes.

Hasson, N., & Joffe, V. (2007). The case for Dynamic Assessment in speech and language therapy. *Child Language Teaching and Therapy*, 23(1), 9–25. https://doi.org/10.1177/0265659007072142

Hasson, N. (2017). *The dynamic assessment of language learning*. London: Routledge. https://doi.org/10.4324/9781315175423

Haug, T. (2011). *Adaptation and evaluation of a German Sign Language test – A computer-based receptive skills test for deaf children ages 4–8 years old*. Hamburg: Hamburg University Press. <http://hup.sub.uni-hamburg.de/purl/HamburgUP_Haug_Adaption>

Haug, T. (2015). Use of information and communication technologies in sign language test development: results of an international survey. *Deafness & Education International* 27(1), 33–38. https://doi.org/10.1179/1557069X14Y.0000000041

Haug, T., & Mann, W. (2008). Adapting tests of sign language assessment to other sign languages – A review of linguistic, cultural, and psychometric problems. *Journal of Deaf Studies and Deaf Education* 13(1), 138–147. https://doi.org/10.1093/deafed/enm027

Hauser, P., Supalla, T., & Bavelier, D. (2008). American Sign Language sentence reproduction test: Development and implications. In R. Müller de Quadros (Ed.), *Sign languages: Spinning and unraveling the past, present and future* (pp. 160–172). Florianopolis, Brazil: Editora Arara Azul.

Haywood, H. C., & Wingenfeld, S. A. (1992). Interactive assessment as a research tool. *The Journal of Special Education* 26(3), 253–268. https://doi.org/10.1177/002246699202600303

Herman, R. (1998a) The need for an assessment of deaf children's signing skills. *Deafness & Education* 22(3), 3–7.

Herman, R. (1998b). Issues in designing an assessment of British Sign Language development. *Proceedings of the conference of the Royal College of Speech & Language Therapists*, 332–337.

Herman, R. (2015). Language assessment in deaf learners. In H. Knoors & M. Marschark (Eds.), *Educating deaf learners: Creating a global evidence base* (pp. 197–212). Oxford: University Press. https://doi.org/10.1093/acprof:oso/9780190215194.003.0009

Herman, R., & Curtin, M. (2017) The BSL Receptive Skills Test: How much has changed in 18 years? Paper presented at the National Conference of the Royal College of Speech & Language Therapists, Glasgow.

Herman, R., Grove, N., Holmes, S., Morgan, G., Sutherland, H., & Woll, B. (2004). *Assessing BSL development: Production Test (Narrative Skills)*. London: City University Publication.

Herman, R., Holmes, S., & Woll, B. (1999). *Assessing British Sign Language development: Receptive Skills Test*. Coleford: Forest Book Services.

Herman, R., Rowley, K., Mason, K., & Morgan, G. (2014). Deficits in narrative abilities in child British Sign Language users with specific language impairment. *International Journal of Language and Communication Disorders* 49(3), 343–353. https://doi.org/10.1111/1460-6984.12078

Herman, R., Rowley, K., & Woll, B. (2015). *Online BSL Receptive Skills Test (RST)*. <https://dcalportal.org/tests>

Herman, R., & Woll, B. (1998). Design and standardisation of an assessment of British Sign Language development for use with young deaf children: Final report for London Regional Office.

Hoskin, J. H. (2017). *Language Therapy in British Sign Language: A study exploring the use of therapeutic strategies and resources by Deaf adults working with young people who have language learning difficulties in British Sign Language (BSL)* (Unpublished PhD dissertation). University College London.

Huberty, T. J., & Koeler, J. R. (1984). A test of the learning potential hypothesis with hearing and deaf students. *The Journal of Educational Research* 78(1), 22–28. https://doi.org/10.1080/00220671.1984.10885566

Johnson, R. E., Liddell, S. K., & Erting, C. J. (1989). Unlocking the curriculum: Principles for achieving access in deaf education. *Gallaudet Research Institute Working Papers* 59(3). Washington, DC: Gallaudet University.

Johnston, T. (2004) The assessment and achievement of proficiency in a native sign language within a sign bilingual program: The pilot Auslan Receptive Skills Test. *Deafness & Education International* 6(2), 57–81. https://doi.org/10.1179/146431504790560582

Kapantzoglou, M., Restrepo, M. A., & Thompson, M. S. (2012). Dynamic assessment of word learning skills: Identifying language impairment in bilingual children. *Language, Speech, and Hearing Services in Schools* 43(1), 81–96. https://doi.org/10.1044/0161-1461(2011/10-0095)

Katz, M. A., & Buchholz, E. S. (1984). Use of the LPAD for cognitive enrichment of a deaf child. *School Psychology Review* 13, 99–106.

Keating, E., & Mirus, G. (2004). American Sign Language in virtual space: Interactions between deaf users of computer-mediated video communication and the impact of technology on language practices. *Language in Society* 32(5), 693–714.

Kiernan, C. Reid, B., & Jones, L. (1982). *Signs and symbols: Use of non-vocal communication systems*. London: Heinemann Educational.

Kyle, J. G. (1987). *Sign & School.* Clevedon: Multilingual Matters.

Lauchlan, F., & Carrigan, D. (2013). *Improving learning through dynamic assessment: A practical classroom resource.* London: Jessica Kingsley Publishers.

Lidz, C. S. (1987). *Dynamic assessment: An interactional approach to evaluating learning potential.* New York, NY: Guilford Press.

Lidz, C. S. (1991). *Practitioner's guide to dynamic assessment.* New York, NY: Guilford Press.

Lidz, C. S (2004). Successful application of a dynamic assessment procedure with deaf students between the ages of four and eight years. *Educational and Child Psychology* 21(1), 59–73.

Mayer, M. (1969). Frog, where are you? New York: Dial Press.

Mann, W. (2009). What can deaf children's vocabulary tell us? The British Sign Language Vocabulary Test. *British Deaf News*, 16–17.

Mann, W. (2018). Measuring deaf learners' language progress in school. In M. Marschark & H. Knoors (Eds.), *Evidence-based practice in deaf education.* Oxford: Oxford University Press.

Mann, W., Da Peña, E., & Morgan, G. (2014). Exploring the use of dynamic language assessment with deaf children, who use American Sign Language: Two case studies. *Journal of Communication Disorders* 52, 16–30. https://doi.org/10.1016/j.jcomdis.2014.05.002

Mann, W., & Haug, T. (2016). New directions in sign language assessment. In M. Marschark & P. Spencer (Eds.), *The Oxford handbook of deaf studies in language* (pp. 299–310). New York, NY: Oxford University Press.

Mann, W., & Marshall, C. (2012). Investigating deaf children's vocabulary knowledge in British Sign Language. *Language Learning* 62(4), 24–51. https://doi.org/10.1111/j.1467-9922.2011.00670.x

Mann, W., Peña, E. D., & Morgan, G. (2015). Child modifiability as a predictor of language abilities in deaf children who use *American Sign Language.* 64(3), 374–385.

Mann, W., Roy, P., & Morgan, G. (2016). Adaptation of a vocabulary test from British Sign Language to American Sign Language. *Language Testing* 33(1), 3–22. https://doi.org/10.1177/0265532215575627

Marchman, V. A., & Fernald, A. (2008). Speed of word recognition and vocabulary knowledge in infancy predict cognitive and language outcomes in later childhood. *Developmental Science* 11, F9–F16. https://doi.org/10.1111/j.1467-7687.2008.00671.x

Marshall, C., Mason, K., Rowley, K., Herman, R., Atkinson, J., Woll, B., & Morgan, G. (2014). Sentence repetition in deaf children with specific language impairment in British Sign Language. *Language Learning and Development* 11(3), 237–251. https://doi.org/10.1080/15475441.2014.917557

Mayberry, R. I., Hall, M. L., & Zvaigzne, M. (2013). Subjective frequency ratings for 432 ASL signs. *Behavior Research Methods* 46(2), 526–539. https://doi.org/10.3758/s13428-013-0370-x

McNeill, D. (1992). *Hand and mind.* Chicago, IL: University of Chicago Press.

Meuris, K., Maes, B., & Zink, I. (2015). Teaching adults with intellectual disability manual signs through their support staff: a key word signing program. *American Journal of Speech-Language Pathology* 24, 545–560. https://doi.org/10.1044/2015_AJSLP-14-0062

Morgan, P. L., Farkas, G., Hillemeier, M. M., Hammer, C. S., & Maczuga, S. (2015.) 24-month-old children with larger oral vocabularies display greater academic and behavioral functioning at kindergarten entry. *Child Development* 86, 1351–1370. https://doi.org/10.1111/cdev.12398

Newell, W., Caccamise, F., Boardman, K., & Holcomb, B. R. (1983). Adaptation of the Language Proficiency Interview (LPI) for assessing sign communicative competence. *Sign Language Studies* 41, 311–352. https://doi.org/10.1353/sls.1983.0012

Ochs, E., & Capps, L. (2001). *Living narrative: Creating lives in everyday storytelling*. Cambridge, MA: Harvard University Press.

Olswang, L. B., & Bain, B. A. (1996). Assessment information for predicting upcoming change in language production. *Journal of Speech & Hearing Research* 39(2), 414–423. https://doi.org/10.1044/jshr.3902.414

Peña, E. D., Iglesias, A. & Lidz, C. S. (2001). Reducing test bias through dynamic assessment of children's word learning ability. *American Journal of Speech-Language Pathology*. 10:138–154.

Peña, E. D., Gillam, R. B., & Bedore, L. M. (2014). Dynamic assessment of narrative ability in English accurately identifies language impairment in English language learners. *Journal of Speech, Language, and Hearing Research* 57(6), 2208–2220. https://doi.org/10.1044/2014_JSLHR-L-13-0151

Peña, E. D., Gillam, R. B., Malek, M., Ruiz-Felter, R., Resendiz, M., Fiestas, C., & Sabel, T. (2006). Dynamic assessment of school-age children's narrative ability: An experimental investigation of classification accuracy. *Journal of Speech, Language, and Hearing Research* 49(5), 1037–1057. https://doi.org/10.1044/1092-4388(2006/074)

Peña, E. D., Reséndiz, M., & Gillam, R. B. (2007). The role of clinical judgements of modifiability in the diagnosis of language impairment. *Advances in Speech Language Pathology* 9(4), 332–345. https://doi.org/10.1080/14417040701413738

Peña, E. D., & Villarreal, B. (2000). Modifiability observation form. Unpublished instrument.

Pickersgill, M., & Gregory, S. (1998). *Sign Bilingualism*. Kimpton: LASER Publications.

Rombouts, E., Maes, B., & Zink, I. (2017). Maintenance of key word signing in adults with intellectual disabilities: Novel signed turns facilitated by partners' consistent input and sign imitation. *Augmentative and Alternative Communication* 33, 121–130. https://doi.org/10.1080/07434618.2017.1326066

Rudd, H., Grove, N., & Pring, T. (2007). Teaching productive sign modifications to children with intellectual impairments. *Augmentative and Alternative Communication* 23, 154–163. https://doi.org/10.1080/07434610601124867

Samuels, C. (2007). 'Universal Design' concept pushed for education. EBSCO Professional Development Collection. <http://www.cflparents.org/information/resources/Systemic-Change/Universal%20Design-Education-Week-07.pdf >

SAASLA LLC. (2015). Unpublished test and web site. San Francisco State University. <https://saasla.com/>

Schieffelin, B. B., & Ochs, E. (Eds.) (1986). *Language socialization across cultures*. Cambridge: Cambridge University Press.

Stinson, M. (2010). In M. Marschark & P. E. Spencer (Eds.), *The Oxford handbook of deaf studies, Vol. 2: Language and Education* (pp. 93–110), New York, NY: Oxford University Press.

Stefánsdóttir, G., & Traustadóttir, R. (2015). Life histories as counter-narratives against dominant and negative stereotypes about people with intellectual disabilities. *Disability & Society* 30, 368–380. https://doi.org/10.1080/09687599.2015.1024827

Tzuriel, D., & Caspri, N. (1992). Cognitive modifiability and cognitive performance of deaf and hard of hearing preschool children. *Journal of Special Education* 26(3), 235–252. https://doi.org/10.1177/002246699202600302

Ukrainetz, T., Harpell, S., Walsh, C., & Coyle, C. (2000). A preliminary investigation of dynamic assessment with Native American kindergartners. *Language, Speech and Hearing Services in Schools* 31, 142–154. https://doi.org/10.1044/0161-1461.3102.142

Valmaseda, M., Pérez, M., Herman, R., Ramírez, N. & Montero, I. (2013). Evaluación de la Competencia Gramatical en LSE: Proceso de Adaptación del BSL-Receptive Skill Test (Test de Habilidades Receptivas). Paper presented at the Congreso del Centro de Normalizacion Linguistica de la Lengua de Signos Espanola, Madrid. <http://www.cnlse.es/sites/default/files/Evaluacion%20de%20la%20competencia%20gra>

Van den Broek-Laven, A., Boers, E., & Van den Bogaerde, B. (2014). Determining aspects of text difficulty for the Sign Language of the Netherlands (NGT) Functional Assessment instrument. *Papers in Language Testing and Assessment – Special Issue* 1, 53–75.

von Tetzchner, S., & Basil, C. (2011). Terminology and notation in written representations of conversations with augmentative and alternative communication. *Augmentative and Alternative Communication* 27, 141–149. https://doi.org/10.3109/07434618.2011.610356

Vygotsky, L. S. (1978). *Mind in society: The development of higher mental process.* Cambridge, MA: Harvard University Press.

Takei, W. (2012). Development of teaching materials to facilitate independence. Paper presented at the 11th Asia Pacific Congress on Deafness, Singapore.

Takei, W. (2016). Assessing Japanese Sign Language vocabulary development of Deaf children. Paper presented at the 12th Asia Pacific Congress of Deafness, Christchurch, New Zealand.

Waite, M. C., Theodoros, D. G., Russell, T. G., & Cahill, L. M. (2010). Internet-based telehealth assessment of language using the CELF-4. *Language Speech & Hearing Services in Schools* 41(4), 445–458. https://doi.org/10.1044/0161-1461

Woll, B., & Barnett, S. (1998). Toward a sociolinguistic perspective on augmentative and alternative communication. *Augmentative and Alternative Communication* 14, 200–211. https://doi.org/10.1080/07434618123312/8376

Woll, B., & Grove, N. (1996) On language deficits and modality in children with Down Syndrome: A case study of twins bilingual in BSL and English. *Journal of Deaf Studies and Deaf Education* 1(4), 271–278. https://doi.org/10.1093/oxfordjournals.deafed.a014302

Woolfe T., Herman R., Roy P., & Woll B. (2010). Early vocabulary development in deaf native signers: A British Sign Language adaptation of the communicative development inventories. *Journal of Child Psychology and Psychiatry* 51(3), 322–331. https://doi.org/10.1111/j.1469-7610.2009.02151.x

CHAPTER 5

Atypical sign language development

Chloë Marshall, Katherine Rowley, Joanna Atkinson,
Tanya Denmark, Joanna Hoskins and Jechil Sieratzki

A major theme in Bencie Woll's research has been what the study of sign
language and atypical signers who have neurological differences can teach
us about language and cognition more generally. In this chapter, we focus on
the growing literature relating to atypical sign language development, with an
emphasis on Bencie's pioneering work in this field. We show that by studying
atypical users of language we gain insights into language and cognitive processes
that would not be obtained by studying typical users, or by limiting research
to spoken languages. We review developmental research of individuals and
groups with Landau-Kleffner Syndrome, Williams Syndrome, Autism Spectrum
Disorder and Specific Language Impairment. Finally, we consider issues relating
to intervention.

0. Setting the scene

Bencie Woll's contribution to research in the area of atypical sign language development cannot be overstated, and her influence on the work described in this
chapter has been profound. She has not only posed, and stimulated colleagues
to pose, new and interesting questions, but she also had a vision of creating the
right conditions for a new generation of Deaf researchers to emerge in British
academia. For example, in 1993, she pioneered Deaf people's access to higher
education by setting up a new support service at Bristol University, where she was
based (see foreword by Jim Kyle, this volume). She founded the "Access for Deaf
Students" initiative, which enabled students to access teaching via sign language
interpreters and new verbatim speech-to-text technology developed as a direct
result of her research collaboration with the Royal National Institute for the Deaf.
Joanna Atkinson was one of the first of these degree students to receive support
from the new centre. It was the start of a fruitful collaboration between Bencie
and Joanna, who together went on to study atypical sign language in signers with

https://doi.org/10.1075/tilar.25.05mar
© 2020 John Benjamins Publishing Company

stroke, autism, specific language impairment, dementia and schizophrenia. Later, when the Deafness, Cognition and Language (DCAL) research centre launched at UCL in 2005, one of its four research strands was with Gary Morgan and Ros Herman on atypical language: Chloë Marshall, Tanya Denmark, Kathryn Mason and Deaf researcher Kate Rowley joined the team working on this strand. In what follows, we discuss some of the work on atypical sign language development that Bencie has inspired and collaborated on with both Deaf and hearing researchers.

A major theme in Bencie's research has been what the study of sign language and atypical signers who have neurological differences can teach us about language and cognition more generally. In this chapter, we focus on the growing literature relating to atypical sign language development, with an emphasis on Bencie's pioneering work and contribution to research in this field. We review studies showing that by studying atypical users of sign language we gain insights into language structure and cognitive processes that would not be obtained by studying only typical users, or by limiting research to only spoken languages. We offer an overview of developmental research in individual and small group sign language studies in Landau-Kleffner Syndrome, Williams Syndrome, Autism Spectrum Disorder and Specific Language Impairment. We end the chapter by considering issues relating to interventions for these groups of individuals.

1.   Introduction

Language development is a robust phenomenon: children all over the world learn their first language with remarkable speed and ease (Pinker, 1994). However, this is not the case for all children. As other authors explore in this volume (Chapter 2, Harris & Clibbens, and Chapter 6, Lillo-Martin, Tsimpli & Smith), deaf children's language acquisition is usually more complicated than that of hearing children. First, the most accessible language for them is generally a sign language, but few deaf children have sign language input early in life (Mitchell & Karchmer, 2004), and this delay influences how successful first sign language acquisition will be. Although access to spoken language through cochlear implantation is improving, many deaf children still have delayed spoken language acquisition (Chapter 1 Morgan, this volume).

Yet it is not just deaf children who can suffer delayed language acquisition – hearing children can too, for reasons endogenous and exogenous to the child. By "endogenous" we mean factors that lie within the child, e.g., learning difficulties such as specific language impairment, autism, down syndrome and Williams syndrome (Marshall, 2013). By "exogenous" we mean factors in the child's environment, such as poor quality and low quantity of input (Roy & Chiat, 2013).

Also, both factors might be at play in the same child. Thinking about the reasons for delayed language development within this framework enables us to make predictions about deaf children who are acquiring a sign language – namely, that their language development can be affected not just by exogenous factors (delayed and poor-quality sign language input) but by endogenous factors too. It is those endogenous factors – and how they potentially interact with the language input – that we explore in this chapter. Specifically, we ask how developmental disorders affect sign language development in deaf children, but also in hearing individuals who are learning a sign language, where this is relevant. Some of the research we discuss necessarily takes the form of single case studies, while other work involves small groups of children.

2. Sign Language acquisition in Landau-Kleffner Syndrome (LKS)

LKS is a severe neurological disorder that affects language abilities, attention and behaviour, begins in childhood, and can evolve into an acquired global aphasia. After a seemingly normal early language development, affected children lose the ability to understand and subsequently to produce spoken language (Landau & Kleffner, 1957). LKS is associated with – or caused by – epilepsy. On electroen-cephalography, typical bilateral temporo-parietal abnormalities occur, particularly during sleep. Clinical seizures are limited. The epilepsy often does not respond well to medical and surgical treatment but usually subsides at puberty. Bencie Woll, to-gether with Harry (Jechil) Sieratzki, a paediatrician, and other colleagues, under-took extensive linguistic and fMRI studies on SC, a 26-year-old left-handed male affected by LKS since the age of 5 years. This fascinating case study (Sieratzki et al., 2001) produced fundamentally new insights into LKS and language development.

SC was profoundly aphasic in English but had good communication skills in British Sign Language (BSL), to which he had been introduced at the age of 13 years. His comprehension of spoken language was limited to a small set of familiar words and short phrases with simple word order, and his articulations were un-intelligible except to those who knew him well. However, SC showed a surprising awareness of English homophones. During a picture naming test, he responded to the target picture *wristwatch* correctly in English, then laughingly explained in BSL that the word "watch" can also mean "to see". For the target picture (salad)-*bowl* he explained that the same word is used for throwing in cricket.

SC's reading was too slow for efficient communication. He recognised the graphic pattern of whole words "by eye", without awareness of letter-sound cor-respondences. When using BSL finger-spelling (i.e., the manual alphabet) he would name each letter one by one slowly, unable to co-articulate a whole word in the way that a deaf person would. In another difference to deaf people, SC did not show spontaneous attention to articulatory lip movements: he lacked the phonological skills required to gain access to spoken language through lip-reading (see Kyle, Campbell, & MacSweeney, 2016, for the role of lip-reading in deaf and hearing children).

Sign language was by far SC's most efficient communication modality. He had normal vocabulary but very uneven abilities in BSL grammar. A feature of all known sign languages is that space is used for grammatical purposes. Signed utterances may assign arbitrary spatial locations to express verb relationships between actors or concepts in linguistic or referential signing space. This space bears no relationship to the real-life location actors or objects and so is 'non-topographic' space. In addition to such purely linguistic use of space, sign languages can directly convey spatial relationships, which involve a direct mapping of real-world relationships in language; they have been described as using topographic space. The expression in sign languages of both non-topographic space and topographic space requires linguistic representations, with non-topographic space using spatial relationships to represent abstract relationships, and topographic space appearing to recruit real-world image structure directly.

SC had learned to use the spatial aspects of BSL to express the real-world locations of objects but had very limited use of abstract signing space for syntactic representations. Sieratzki et al. (2001) speculated that this pattern reflected an inability to access Broca's area without the gateway of an intact auditory speech cortex. To investigate SC's language processing in more detail, they conducted fMRI studies during various language tasks. When hearing words, SC showed very strong bilateral temporo-parietal activation, greater in the right hemisphere than left, including Broca's area. This lateralisation pattern matched SC's epileptic focus in childhood and right-hemispheric dominance for language. When viewing faces mouthing numbers, only the cingulate was activated (indicating attention), without the auditory cortex (consistent with SC's inability to lip-read). When viewing written words, there was non-continuous and non-robust activation of Broca's area and auditory cortex. This activation was mostly only in the left hemisphere without the supramarginal gyrus and posterior association cortices (areas involved in letter-sound conversion and retrieval), correlating with reading or recognition of words as fixed graphic patterns (which is a non-dominant hemisphere skill).

SC might have been using the capacity of the visual cortex to analyse temporal changes in spatial patterning as a substitute route for decoding sign language. The way SC processed language provides a neuro-linguistic argument as to why children with LKS should be given the opportunity to learn a natural sign language (Woll & Sieratzki, 1996) and shows how human language can function without access to its primary processing system.

3. Sign language acquisition in Williams syndrome

The earliest collaboration between Joanna Atkinson and Bencie Woll focused on a unique case of a deaf person with specific visuospatial developmental learning disabilities that were similar in nature to Williams Syndrome (Atkinson, Woll, & Gathercole, 2002). At the time, Ursula Bellugi's lab in San Diego was publishing both ground-breaking research into the relationship between language and visuospatial cognition in Williams syndrome (e.g., Bellugi et al., 2000) and equally impressive work on American Deaf signers with either sign language aphasias after left-hemisphere strokes or visuospatial impairments after right-hemisphere strokes (e.g., Poizner et al., 1987). There was great interest in the research community at that time in the relationship between the development of language and cognition, especially where dissociations could be seen between them. Language and cognition were often described in terms of separate modules within the brain within the framework of the modularity hypothesis (Pinker, 1994), so there was interest in trying to find cases where impairments in one domain affected function in another, in order to provide evidence in support of, or against, modularity.

Williams syndrome, a rare congenital disorder characterised by relatively preserved language but marked difficulties with visuospatial cognition, had been extensively studied in hearing people but no one had been able to study this pattern in a born deaf user of a signed, rather than spoken, language. The case of 30 year-old 'Heather' was particularly interesting because she was similar to the characteristic phenotype of Williams syndrome in physical appearance and cognitive abilities, but was also congenitally deaf and a user of BSL. The existence of sign space as grammatical feature in sign languages afforded a unique opportunity to study the interface between language and visuospatial cognition. Impaired visuospatial cognition might be more negative for language development and processing in BSL than in any spoken language. Heather offered the first opportunity to explore the consequences of specific visuospatial developmental learning difficulties on the linguistic system when the language used is visual and spatial, with the prediction that the consequences of visuospatial cognitive impairments might be particularly severe for sign languages.

Heather was born to hearing parents and is therefore a non-native signer with delayed BSL acquisition, but she was educated from a young age using BSL. She showed a preference for BSL over sign-supported English (SSE) in general conversation and her difficulties could not be explained by a lack of proficiency in BSL, or a preference for SSE. Assessments revealed a large vocabulary in BSL, and overall presented a picture of relative competence in BSL grammar, with language abilities well in advance of her impaired visuospatial cognition. However, she did show specific deficits in those areas of BSL which directly rely on spatial representations for linguistic purposes i.e., verb agreement and referential indices. There was also evidence of an impaired ability to use topographical space. During narrative tasks, Heather failed to maintain topographic relationships when using grammatical devices such as spatial and agreement verbs. She did not use pronominal reference or role shift to mark the spatial relationships between story protagonists. By contrast, linguistic devices which do not incorporate spatial relationships, such as noun-verb distinctions and negation, were preserved. Comprehension and production of spatialized syntax (i.e. agreement verbs) was also relatively intact in tests of single sentences where space is used only to show grammatical relationships. However, Heather displayed marked problems with agreement verbs in the narrative test, as agreement verbs in context must inflect to agree not only with the person but also with topographic locations established in earlier sentences in the narrative. Thus, all areas of grammar that require the use of topographic space were compromised.

The learning of a visuospatial language, therefore, is not in itself dependent on intact visuospatial cognition (see the description of Christopher in Morgan, Woll, Tsimpli, & Smith, 2002 and Chapter 6 this volume). However, the pattern of breakdown in BSL abilities revealed a dissociation within BSL grammar between devices that depend on grammatical processes involving space and those that do not. This is highlighted by the example of plurals. In BSL, plurals can either be marked by following the noun with a classifier and distributive movement, or – in a construction which is not incorrect but is atypical – by a lexical quantifier (MANY) following the noun. Heather showed a clear preference for the latter device, which does not rely on spatial relationships to express grammatical meaning.

There are interesting similarities and differences between Heather's signing and that of the signers who had visuospatial impairments following right hemisphere damage and who were studied by Poizner and colleagues (Hickok et al., 1999; Poizner et al., 1987; Poizner & Kegl, 1992). Heather's errors at both the sentential and the narrative levels are reminiscent of those found in signers with right hemisphere damage, and yet, unlike them, she exhibited a full range of affective and grammatical facial expression and normal prosody in spontaneous, everyday communication.

This research was important because it showed that people with visuospatial impairments are still able to use sign language, albeit with subtle impairments to aspects that use topographical space. Often these difficulties would only become apparent in forced-response paradigms because compensatory strategies were used in everyday conversation, such as using a more English-like sign order to get around spatial difficulties.

At the time, there were questions about which aspects of sign language were purely linguistic and which aspects would require intact visuospatial cognition to proceed. This study helped to untangle some of those issues. Inspired by this work, Quinto-Pozos et al. (2013) presented a case study of an adolescent female with average intelligence who had been reported to struggle with spatial aspects of American Sign Language (ASL) as a child. Results of a battery of linguistic tests confirmed that despite relatively good ASL skills overall, she did have specific difficulties on spatial tasks that required attention to ASL and nonlinguistic topographic space or changes in visual perspective, such as classifiers and referential shift. Furthermore, tests of non-linguistic visuospatial cognition suggested that she had some difficulties with visuospatial abilities. Just as Atkinson et al. (2002) proposed for Heather, Quinto-Pozos et al. (2013) suggested that in their case study visuospatial difficulties affected acquisition of those aspects of a sign language that are heavily dependent on visuospatial processing.

Another key feature of signing is that signers must pay attention to the face (see Chapters 2 by Harris & Clibbens and Chapter 3 by Baker & van den Bogaerde, this volume). Attention to the face is particularly challenging in children with autism. How this plays out in a context where a child with autism is learning to sign is interesting, and we turn to this topic next.

4.   Sign language acquisition in Autism

Hearing children with autism spectrum disorder (ASD) generally show reduced attention towards faces and have impairments in emotion perception and production of facial expressions (Dawson et al., 2005; MacDonald et al., 1989; Volker et al., 2009). The impairments with facial emotion recognition in hearing children with ASD also extend to vocal emotion recognition (Peppe et al., 2006; Tager-Flusberg, 1981). Prevalence studies have demonstrated that deafness is more common in children with ASD than in children not diagnosed with ASD (e.g., Rosenhall et al., 1999), although it is not clear why this is the case. Yet despite a growing awareness of individuals with a dual diagnosis of deafness and ASD, there have been very few published studies involving this group.

In sign languages, the face is a crucial articulator; facial actions are used to supplement the information on the hands (Roberts & Hindley, 1999). Facial expressions convey the same emotional information (e.g., happiness, surprise, fear) as they do in spoken languages, but they also have linguistic functions. Linguistic facial actions are known as non-manual markers. Non-manual markers are crucial for grammar, because when they are produced in conjunction with a single sign phrase they change the meaning from an assertion, to a question, a statement of negation or a relative clause simply by varying the type of facial action produced (Liddell, 1980).

Given evidence of impairment with facial and vocal emotion recognition during language processing in hearing children with ASD, an obvious avenue for research is to examine whether equivalent difficulties occur in deaf children with ASD and if there is a reduced use of the face during production of BSL. This research, undertaken as a PhD thesis with Joanna Atkinson as a supervisor (Denmark, 2011), was the first to systematically investigate general face-processing ability and the comprehension and production of affective facial expressions and facially-expressed linguistic structures in BSL in deaf children with ASD.

Denmark et al. (2014) investigated facial expression recognition in 13 severely-profoundly deaf children and young people with ASD (aged 9–17 years) and a control group of non-ASD deaf participants matched for age, non-verbal reasoning and BSL skills. Only one child in each group was a native signer and had deaf parents, but all children were able to produce phrases in BSL. Participants were shown video clips of signed sentences produced with different emotions in two conditions (masked – where the face was covered but the hands were still visible; unmasked – where the face was visible, as were the hands). The ASD group was less accurate in their judgments of emotion compared to the non-ASD group. Moreover, the significant interaction between group (ASD versus non-ASD) and condition (masked vs. unmasked) showed that whereas masking the face impaired both groups, the effect was significantly greater for the non-ASD group than the ASD group.

In a further study (Denmark et al., 2019), both groups were compared on their production of affective facial expressions during a BSL narrative task (The BSL Production Test, Herman et al., 2004; see Chapter 4). Non-ASD deaf children produced facial expressions which were closely aligned with those of the story protagonists in the video. In contrast, the ASD group produced fewer targeted expressions and showed qualitative differences in the facial actions that they did produce. This finding is consistent with the finding of impairments in the production of signals of emotion in hearing groups with ASD (MacDonald et al., 1989; Volker et al., 2009).

Additionally, both groups were compared on their comprehension and production of linguistic facial expressions (see Denmark, 2011, for more detail). For example, Atkinson et al.'s (2004) Negation Test was adapted to measure the comprehension and production of negation facial markers in BSL. Furthermore, the use of questions and adverbials – which again are expressed on the face – was also explored in separate studies using similar methodologies. These studies focusing on linguistic uses of the face demonstrated general preservation of facial actions in BSL, which hold a purely linguistic function, with the notable exception of adverbials. It was hypothesised based on these findings that adverbial facial expressions caused more difficulty for the deaf ASD group because they require attributions about the mental state of others, i.e., Theory of Mind (Brownwell & Martino, 1998; Smith et al., 2003).

These studies are the first to compare both deaf children with ASD and TD deaf children on their use of affective and linguistic facial expressions in sign language. The results suggest that deaf individuals with ASD are not generally impaired with face processing; rather they have a highly specific and subtle pattern of impairments with using the face in sign language. Their BSL production and receptive skills did not differ significantly from those of non-ASD deaf controls of the same age, suggesting their grammar was comparable, and they had broad preservation of facial actions in BSL which hold a purely linguistic function. However, like hearing people with ASD, deaf signers with ASD appear to have a primary deficit in emotional reasoning and Theory of Mind.

Denmark's findings support Shield's (2010, p. 2) notion that "sign language forces learners to employ cognitive skills thought to be impaired in autism", and suggest that the attention to faces required by signed communication may prevent more substantial face processing impairments arising in children with ASD. However, in order to separate effects of deafness and sign language use on individuals with ASD, investigation of hearing individuals with ASD who use sign language is warranted. With the exception of a study of a hearing savant who learnt BSL in adulthood (Smith et al., 2011; see Chapter 6 this volume), there have been no other known studies to date that have explored how hearing individuals with ASD acquire a sign language.

5. Sign language acquisition in Specific Language Impairment (SLI)

It is well documented that seven percent of the hearing population has Specific Language Impairment (SLI), a disorder that affects the development of language (Norbury et al., 2016; Tomblin et al., 1997). Traditionally, SLI was defined as occurring despite having normal non-verbal intelligence, hearing, cognitive and motoric functions; however, the specificity of SLI to language is now under debate due to high levels of co-morbidity with other disorders such as dyslexia and autism (see Bishop et al., 2017, who suggest that the term "Developmental Language Disorder" might be more appropriate). Studies of SLI across a large number of languages have demonstrated that it is heterogeneous: it can have an impact on one or more aspects of language, i.e., phonology, morphology, syntax and semantics, and it can affect both receptive and productive language (Leonard, 1998). Deaf children have traditionally been excluded from studies of SLI because hearing loss is strongly associated with delays in the development of spoken languages. However, there is no reason for hearing loss to have an impact on the acquisition of sign languages.

Indeed, recent studies have demonstrated that deaf children learning a sign language *can* have a language-learning disorder that occurs in addition to their deafness (Morgan et al., 2007; Mason et al., 2010; Quinto-Pozos et al., 2011). Despite the difference in modality, spoken and sign languages share many similar linguistic features and are processed in similar ways (Emmorey, 2002). Additionally, many studies have found that the developmental patterns of spoken and sign languages are remarkably similar (Petitto & Marentette, 1991; Chen-Pichler, 2012). As spoken and sign languages are acquired and processed in similar ways, it stands to reason that disorders such as SLI can impact the acquisition of sign language in deaf children. However, identifying SLI in sign language is challenging for several reasons (Herman et al., 2014). As 90–95% of deaf children are born to hearing parents (Mitchell & Karchmer, 2004), many deaf children have impoverished access to a fluent model of sign language. This means that many deaf children have delayed language, and it is very challenging to tease apart language delay and language disorder. Additionally, hearing children with SLI have been found to use gestures in order to compensate for their difficulties with language (Wray et al., 2017), but in sign language users it can be difficult to distinguish between gestures and signs (Goldin-Meadow, 2003), especially for parents and professionals who are not fluent in sign language.

Despite these challenges, researchers have found ways to assess and identify language impairments in sign language (see the discussion of language assessment in Chapter 4, this volume). Indeed, it was the development of sign language assessments, together with the work by Bencie Woll and colleagues investigating how sign language could be impaired in different populations (including the case studies of Landau-Kleffner Syndrome and Williams syndrome described earlier in this chapter), that led to a point where researchers could tackle the potentially more complex question of SLI in sign.

In the UK, several deaf signing children were referred to the Compass Centre at City University London (Herman et al., 2014) to undergo language and cognitive assessments because of concerns with their language development, and it was clear from these assessments that some had language-learning problems in addition their deafness. One case study reported that a deaf child of deaf signing parents had delayed BSL acquisition despite regular exposure to fluent BSL from birth (Morgan et al., 2007). Because this delay could not be explained by impoverished access to BSL, the researchers concluded that this child had a language disorder that impacted his BSL development (Morgan et al., 2007).

To follow up on this case study, a larger-scale study was conducted to assess and identify SLI in BSL, as well as to determine the prevalence of SLI in BSL (Mason et al., 2010). Initially, a screening questionnaire was formulated based on characteristics of SLI identified in studies of spoken language (Leonard, 1998). In addition to determining which characteristics of SLI each child displayed, background information such as degree of hearing loss, education placement, age of sign language acquisition, pre-existing conditions, access to fluent sign language models etc. were also included in this pre-screening questionnaire. This questionnaire was sent out to 72 schools across the U.K., which included mainstreams and deaf schools. 50 questionnaires were returned and of the 50 deaf children referred, 30 deaf children were tested (16 males, aged 5 to 15 years, mean age = 11.5 years). Out of these 30, 13 were confirmed to have language delay despite sufficient exposure to BSL and normal cognitive and motoric functions (Mason et al., 2010). Mason et al. (2010) calculated that this amounts to around 6.4% of the deaf signing population. If accurate, this estimate suggests a similar prevalence of SLI in speaking and signing children.

Standardised tests of BSL comprehension (BSL Receptive Skills Test, Herman et al., 1999) and production (BSL Production Task, Herman et al., 2004) were used to determine whether or not the children's receptive or productive language was within the levels expected for their age. All children were found to have delayed receptive or productive language, or both. To assess non-verbal cognition, three subtests of the British Ability Scales were used (Matrices, Pattern Construction and Recall of Design), and all 13 children scored age-appropriately. Motor dexterity was assessed using a bead-threading task, and none of the children exhibited difficulties with fine motor control. By ruling out cognitive and motoric deficits, the children's difficulties with language were thus attributed to SLI (Mason et al., 2010).

Further measures were used to assess which areas of language these 13 children had difficulties with in order to identify possible characteristics of SLI in BSL. Sentence repetition tasks have been used as one of the measures to identify SLI in hearing children and poor performance on this test is a good indicator of SLI in hearing children (Conti-Ramsden et al., 2001). As explained earlier, SLI can impact phonology, morphology, syntax, semantics, and sentence repetition can test those aspects of language. To further characterise SLI in BSL, a BSL sentence repetition test was created and administered. A subset of 11 deaf children in the SLI group were compared to age-matched controls and the SLI group performed significantly worse on this test (Marshall et al., 2015). The SLI group achieved lower accuracy scores overall and were more likely to drop lexical items, facial expressions and verb morphological structures. They also were less likely to produce sentences using the correct sign order or convey the correct overall meaning (Marshall et al., 2015). Sentence repetition tests are thus likely to be a robust measure for identifying SLI in BSL, as in spoken languages (see also Chapter 4, Herman et al., on the use of similar tests with adult learners of sign language to assess proficiency).

However, not all tests that are sensitive to SLI in hearing children seem to be so effective at identifying signers with SLI. The Nonsense Sign Repetition Test (Mann et al., 2010) was used to test short-term phonological working memory by asking children to repeat nonsense signs presented to them on a computer screen. For spoken languages, nonword repetition tasks are found to be a robust measure to identify SLI in hearing children (Gathercole & Baddeley, 1990); however, for BSL the Nonsense Sign Repetition Test does not seem to have the same sensitivity as only 4 of the 13 children achieved below-average scores (Mason et al., 2010). Marshall, Mann and Morgan (2011) argued that this cross-linguistic difference might be due to differences in the phonological structure of signed and spoken languages.

Marshall et al. (2013) administered a semantic fluency task, which requires participants to name as many items as they can in the space of a minute from particular semantic categories such as "animals" and "foods", in order to assess lexical and semantic organisation. There is evidence that some hearing children with SLI name fewer lexical items on semantic fluency tasks compared to typically developing children (e.g., Henry et al., 2012). For this group of deaf children with SLI, there were no differences in the number of lexical items named when comparing them to a control group of deaf children who have age-appropriate language (as determined by the standardised language assessments described earlier). However, a small subset of the group was slow to name items in the first 15 seconds (out of 60 seconds) compared to the control group, and made particular errors, for example the creation of non-existing compound forms ("redberry") and circumlocutions ("mouse in wheel, you know"), which suggests the presence of lexical retrieval difficulties in these children (Marshall et al., 2013).

The findings reported above confirm the existence of SLI in deaf children who sign, and this has both theoretical and practical implications. This research provides new insights into how different theories can be applied to atypical language development in a different modality. Previous research on SLI did not consider sign language when formulating theories of possible causes of SLI, some of which cannot account for SLI in sign languages (e.g. rapid auditory processing deficits, Tallal, 2000; see Mason et al., 2010; and Herman et al., 2014, for further discussion). Additionally, this research has given us a way to assess and identify SLI in deaf children who sign. This has important implications for practitioners who need to be aware that some deaf children who sign may have language deficits that cannot be attributed to their deafness. In such cases, further and specialised assessments will be needed in order to diagnose SLI.

There is still much to be researched in deaf signers with SLI. Firstly, none have been studied over a period of time, so we have no idea whether their language difficulties get more severe as they get older or whether they catch up with their typically-developing deaf peers. We know from the research literature on spoken

SLI that there is likely to be wide variation in outcomes but that a significant pro-portion of individuals will have lasting impairments (Clegg et al., 2004; Durkin et al., 2015). What that variation looks like for sign SLI, and what factors predict that variation, are things we currently do not understand. Secondly, the majority of research on sign SLI has been carried out in BSL. Although research groups in other countries are beginning to identify SLI in their sign languages (e.g. Quinto-Pozos, Singleton, & Hauser, 2017, for ASL; Bogliotti, Puissant-Schontz, & Marshall, 2017, for French Sign Language), we do not yet know whether it will have the same characteristics in those languages, although we predict that it will look very similar. And thirdly, we don't yet know what interventions can success-fully support sign language learning in children with sign SLI. Nevertheless, we turn to intervention studies now, to survey initial work in this area.

6.   Intervention studies with deaf children who have impairments in their acquisition of sign language

Researchers have identified the need for assessment tools and for practitioners specifically trained to meet the needs of deaf children who use sign languages and have language learning difficulties (See Chapter 4, this volume). The number of studies that have explored the use of interventions is few (in contrast to the extensive research literature on speech and language therapy for deaf children who use spoken language), but it is growing. One approach to intervention is mediated learning, whose activities offer children opportunities to learn and practise new skills with an adult who is able to explain the aim of the activities, and their relevance to the child's life and learning. Mann et al. (2014) explored the use of mediated learning for vocabulary intervention with two deaf children (aged 7 and 8 years) who used ASL. Practitioners found these techniques useful for understanding and supporting children who have difficulties in acquiring ASL, because of their potential to distinguish between disordered language develop-ment and delay. Whilst one of the children was able to move quickly through the mediated learning activities, the other needed more time and repetition to develop skills. The results of this study indicated that children with language difficulties in the signed and spoken modalities respond in a similar way to intervention by trained practitioners.

There have been some attempts to carry out interventions that target deaf children's reported difficulties with Theory of Mind. Wellman and Peterson (2013) carried out an intervention with 43 deaf children (aged 5–13 years) us-ing a program developed for hearing children with autism. The children all used Australian Sign Language, did not have an ASD diagnosis, and had hearing parents.

The 13 children (aged 7 to 13 years) in the Theory of Mind intervention group responded well to the intervention, and the findings were strengthened by the study design which included a control group and a 'non-Theory of Mind' training group, both matched for age. The study also highlights one of many challenges in this area: the researchers did not have direct communication with their deaf child participants but instead worked with sign language interpreters.

Chilton and Beazley (2014) avoided the challenge of using interpreters when working with 10 deaf participants to develop mental state language. Participants were aged from mid-teens to 50s and self-identified as having everyday communication difficulties. Four were BSL users, three used spoken English, and three used a mixture of both languages. The research team adapted their language and communication to meet their participants' needs within the intervention. The study used a language-modified version of the Strange Stories text (Happé, 1994), an intervention previously developed for hearing children with autism using spoken language. Both hearing tutors, a Speech and Language Therapist and a Teacher of the Deaf, provided the intervention. Participant feedback and tutor reflection indicated that intervention was valued by participants, and that adapted materials could be used with people who used sign language.

Novel interventions aimed at improving sign language development have also been studied. Beal-Alvarez and Easterbrooks (2013) evaluated a six-week intervention study based on repeated viewings of ASL stories with scripted teacher mediation to improve the use of complex morphological structures termed 'classifiers'. Although the intervention group was small (10 children, aged 7 to 10 years), and there was no control group, the study showed that children's use of classifiers improved with intervention. Monitoring during non-intervention phases and follow-up after four weeks showed that some children maintained the benefits from intervention. As with Mann et al.'s (2014) study, this intervention focused on a specific language skill and required intense and specific training for the teachers delivering the intervention, in addition to their previous teaching and sign language qualifications. Providing this level of training for staff makes applicability of the interventions to a wider range of language skills or practitioners more difficult due to the availability of time and funding, as well as appropriate trainers and supervisors.

An exploration of the training needs of practitioners who work with deaf children and who are Deaf themselves indicates that providing information about language development, disorder and intervention in sign language is valued by Deaf practitioners as well as by speech and language therapists (Hoskin, 2017). Enabling co-working between these two groups (i.e. Deaf practitioners and hearing speech and language therapists) promoted shared understanding of children's language difficulties in BSL and the possibility of applying intervention strategies.

The study highlights the need for the development of the role of Deaf language practitioner or 'therapist' through training and supervision opportunities.

Taken together, this last piece of research indicates that children and young people with language learning difficulties in sign languages can benefit from assessment and intervention that draws on findings from studies of hearing children with spoken language difficulties. In order to make assessment and intervention approaches more widely available to deaf children, more training and tools are required which provide practitioners with a framework within which to meet the specific language and learning needs of children who use sign language.

7. Conclusions

The study of atypical sign language development has obvious practical implications. Practitioners working with children and young people who use *spoken* language, such as speech and language therapists and specialist teachers, have access to a research base and professional training about typical and atypical language development, and language interventions (Lindsay et al., 2012). Interventions for hearing individuals with language disorders are far in advance of those provided for deaf individuals. There is compelling evidence that hearing children and young people benefit from structured, evidence-based language interventions: these need to be available for deaf signing children and young people too.

The study of atypical sign language development also has important implications for theories of language development and language processing. Investigating sign languages in comparison to spoken languages enables the modality-specific versus modality-general aspects of impaired language to be disentangled, and this in turn offers a new angle on the relationship between language, cognition and sensory processing more generally. At a quite basic level, the fact that SLI is not confined to children learning language in the auditory modality but can also occur in signers supports amodal models of language development and language processing. On the other hand, subtle differences between the language difficulties that characterise SLI in spoken and signed languages (e.g., non-word repetition is problematic for hearing children with SLI in comparison to their typically developing peers, but non-sign repetition does not seem to distinguish signers with and without SLI) suggest there are modality-specific effects on how SLI presents in spoken and signed languages. The data from Heather (Section 3) and from the case study of an adolescent girl reported by Quinto-Pozos et al. (2013) suggest that while a visuospatial difficulty can impact on certain grammatical structures in a sign language, its effects are not very serious: at least some sign language acquisition is possible in cases such as these. Indeed, the work reported in this chapter on individuals with Landau-Kleffner Syndrome (Section 2) and Autism (Section 4) reveals just how robust language-learning can be despite the challenges of these disorders, and that sign language might bring benefits unavailable in spoken language. There is still much to be accomplished with respect to all of these lines of research, but the work discussed in this chapter provides a firm foundation, and a model for how to proceed in sign languages other than BSL.

References

Atkinson, J., Campbell, R., Marshall, J., Thacker, A., & Woll, B. (2004). Understanding 'not': Neuropsychological dissociations between hand and head markers of negation in BSL. *Neuropsychologia* 42, 214–229. https://doi.org/10.1016/S0028-3932(03)00186-6

Atkinson, J. R., Woll, B., & Gathercole, S. (2002). The impact of developmental visuospatial learning difficulties on British Sign Language. *Neurocase* 8, 424–441. https://doi.org/10.1076/neur.8.5.424.16176

Beal-Alvarez, J. S., & Easterbrooks, S. R. (2013). Increasing children's ASL classifier production: a multicomponent intervention. *American Annals of the Deaf* 158, 311–333. https://doi.org/10.1353/aad.2013.0028

Bellugi, U., Lichtenberger, L., Jones, W., Lai, Z., & St George, M. (2000). The neurocognitive profile of Williams Syndrome: A complex pattern of strengths and weaknesses. *Journal of Cognitive Neuroscience* 12, 7–29. https://doi.org/10.1162/089892900561959

Bishop, D. V. M., Snowling, M. J., Thompson, P. A. Greehlagh, T., & the CATALISE-2 Consortium. (2017). Phase 2 of CATALISE: A multinational and multidisciplinary Delphi consensus study of problems with language development: Terminology. *Journal of Child Psychology and Psychiatry* 58, 1068–1080. https://doi.org/10.1111/jcpp.12721

Bogliotti, C., Puissant-Schontz, L., & Marshall, C. R. (2017). L'atypie langagière chez les enfants sourds: Une piste pour définir le développement du langage normal et pathologique dans les langues des signes. In C. Bogliotti, F. Isel, & A. Lacheret-Dujour (Eds.), *Atypie langagière de l'enfance à l'âge adulte* (pp. 75–114). Paris: De Boeck.

Brownwell, H., & Martino, G. (1998). Deficits in inference and social cognition: The effects of right hemisphere brain damage on discourse. In M. Beeman & C. Chiarello (Eds.), *Right hemisphere language comprehension: Perspectives from cognitive neuroscience* (pp. 309–328). Mahwah, NJ: Lawrence Erlbaum Associates.

Chen Pichler, D. (2012). Chapter 29: Language acquisition. In R. Pfau, B. Woll, & M. Steinbach (Eds.), *Handbook of linguistics and communication science: Sign language*. Berlin: De Gruyter.

Chilton, H., & Beazley, S. (2014). Theory of mind: Are there wider implications from working with d/Deaf people? *Disability & Society* 29, 184–197. https://doi.org/10.1080/09687599.2013.816623

Clegg, J., Hollis, C., Mawhood, L., & Rutter, M. (2004). Developmental language disorders – A follow-up in later adult life. Cognitive, language and psychosocial outcomes. *Journal of Child Psychology and Psychiatry* 46, 128–149. https://doi.org/10.1111/j.1469-7610.2004.00342.x

Conti-Ramsden, G., Botting, N., & Faragher, B. (2001). Psycholinguistic markers for specific language impairment (SLI). *Journal of Child Psychology and Psychiatry* 42, 741–748. https://doi.org/10.1111/1469-7610.00770

Dawson, G., Webb, S. J., & McPartland, J. (2005). Understanding the nature of face processing impairment in autism: Insights from behavioural and electrophysiological studies. *Developmental Neuropsychology* 27, 403–424. https://doi.org/10.1207/s15326942dn2703_6

Denmark, T. (2011). *Do deaf children with Autism Spectrum Disorder show deficits in the comprehension and production of emotional and linguistic facial expressions in British Sign Language?* (Unpublished doctoral dissertation). University College London.

Denmark, T., Atkinson, J., Campbell, R., & Swettenham, J. (2014). How do typically developing deaf children and deaf children with Autism Spectrum Disorder use the face when comprehending emotional facial expressions in British Sign Language? *Journal of Autism and Developmental Disorders* 44, 2584–2592. https://doi.org/10.1007/s10803-014-2130-x

Denmark, T., Atkinson, J., Campbell, R., & Swettenham, J. (2019). Signing with the face: Emotional expression in narrative production in deaf children with Autism Spectrum Disorder. *Journal of Autism and Developmental Disorders*, 49, 294–306. https://doi.org/10.1007/s10803-018-3756-x

Durkin, K., Mok, P., &Conti-Ramsden, G. (2015). Core subjects at the end of primary school: identifying and explaining relative strengths of children with specific language impairment (SLI). *International Journal of Language and Communication Disorders* 50, 226–240. https://doi.org/10.1111/1460-6984.12137

Emmorey, K. (2002). *Language, cognition, and the brain: Insights from sign language research.* Mahwah, NJ: Lawrence Erlbaum Associates.

Gathercole, S., & Baddeley, A. (1990). Phonological memory deficits in language disordered children: Is there a causal connection? *Journal of Memory and Language* 29, 336–360. https://doi.org/10.1016/0749-596X(90)90004-J

Goldin-Meadow, S. (2003). *The resilience of language: What gesture creation in deaf children can tell us about how all children learn language.* New York, NY: Psychology Press.

Happé, F. G. (1994). An advanced test of theory of mind: Understanding of story characters' thoughts and feelings by able autistic, mentally handicapped, and normal children and adults. *Journal of Autism and Developmental Disorders* 24, 129–154. https://doi.org/10.1007/BF02172093

Henry, L. A., Messer, D. J., & Nash, G. (2012). Executive functioning in children with specific language impairment. *Journal of Child Psychology and Psychiatry* 53, 37–45. https://doi.org/10.1111/j.1469-7610.2011.02430.x

Herman, R., Grove, N., Holmes, S., Morgan, G., Sutherland, H., & Woll, B. (2004). *Assessing BSL development: Production Test (narrative skills).* London: City University Publication.

Herman, R., Holmes, S., & Woll, B. (1999). *Assessing British Sign Language development: Receptive Skills Test.* Gloucestershire: Forest Bookshop.

Herman, R., Rowley, K., Marshall, C., Mason, K., Atkinson, J., Woll, B., & Morgan, G. (2014). Profiling SLI in deaf children who are sign language users. In D. Quinto-Pozos (Ed.), *Multilingual aspects of signed language communication and disorder* (pp. 45–69). Bristol: Multilingual Matters. https://doi.org/10.21832/9781783091317-005

Hickok, G., Wilson, M., Clark, K., Klima, E. S., Kritchevsky, M., & Bellugi, U. (1999). Discourse deficits following right hemisphere damage in deaf signers. *Brain and Language* 66, 233–248. https://doi.org/10.1006/brln.1998.1995

Hoskin, J. (2017). *Language therapy in BSL: A study exploring the use of therapeutic strategies and resources by deaf adults working with young people who have language learning difficulties in British Sign Language* (Unpublished doctoral dissertation). University College London.

Kyle, F. E., Campbell, R., & MacSweeney, M. (2016). The relative contributions of speechreading and vocabulary to deaf and hearing children's reading ability. *Research in Developmental Disabilities* 48, 13–24. https://doi.org/10.1016/j.ridd.2015.10.004

Landau, W., & Kleffner, F. (1957). Syndrome of acquired aphasia with convulsive disorder in children. *Neurology* 7, 523–530. https://doi.org/10.1212/WNL.7.8.523

Leonard, L. (1998). *Children with Specific Language Impairment.* Cambridge, MA: The MIT Press.

Liddell, S. (1980). *American Sign Language syntax.* The Hague: Mouton.

Lindsay, G., Dockrell, J., Law, J., & Roulstone, S. (2012). *The Better Communication Research Programme: Improving provision for children and young people with speech, language and communication needs,* DFE-RR247-BCRP1, 1–38. London: DfE.

MacDonald, H., Rutter, M., Howlin, P., Rios, P., Le Couteur, A., Evered, C., & Folstein, S. (1989). Recognition and expression of emotional cues by autistic and normal adults. *Journal of Child Psychology and Psychiatry* 30, 865–877. https://doi.org/10.1111/j.1469-7610.1989.tb00288.x

Mann, W., Marshall, C. R., Mason, K., & Morgan, G. (2010). The acquisition of sign language: The impact of phonetic complexity on phonology. *Language Learning and Development* 6, 60–86. https://doi.org/10.1080/15475440903245951

Mann, W., Peña, E. D., & Morgan, G. (2014). Exploring the use of dynamic language assessment with deaf children, who use American Sign Language: Two case studies. *Journal of Communication Disorders* 52, 16–30. https://doi.org/10.1016/j.jcomdis.2014.05.002

Marshall, C. R. (2013). Introduction. In C. R. Marshall (Ed.), *Current Issues in Developmental Disorders* (pp. 1–15). London: Psychology Press.

Marshall, C. R., Mann, W., & Morgan, G. (2011). Short term memory in signed languages: Not just a disadvantage for serial recall. *Frontiers in Psychology* 2,102. https://doi.org/10.3389/fpsyg.2011.00102

Marshall, C. R., Mason, K., Rowley, K., Herman, R., Atkinson, J., Woll, B., & Morgan, G. (2015). Sentence repetition in deaf children with specific language impairment in British Sign Language. *Language Learning and Development* 11, 237–251. https://doi.org/10.1080/15475441.2014.917557

Marshall, C. R., Rowley, K., Mason, K., Herman, R., & Morgan, G. (2013). Lexical organisation in deaf children who use British Sign Language: Evidence from a semantic fluency task. *Journal of Child Language* 40, 193–220. https://doi.org/10.1017/S0305000912000116

Mason, K., Rowley, K., Marshall, C. R., Atkinson, J. R., Herman, R., Woll, B., & Morgan, G. (2010). Identifying SLI in Deaf children acquiring British Sign Language: Implications for theory and practice. *British Journal of Developmental Psychology* 28, 33–49. https://doi.org/10.1348/026151009X484190

Mitchell, R. & Karchmer, M. (2004). Chasing the mystical ten percent: Parental hearing status of deaf and hard of hearing students in the United States. *Sign Language Studies* 4, 138–163. https://doi.org/10.1353/sls.2004.0005

Morgan, G., Herman, R., & Woll, B. (2007). Language impairments in sign language: breakthroughs and puzzles. *International Journal for Language and Communication Disorders* 42, 97–105. https://doi.org/10.1080/13682820600783178

Morgan, G., Woll, B., Tsimpli, I., & Smith, N. V. (2002). The effects of modality on BSL development in an exceptional learner. In R. Meier, K. Cormier, & D. Quinto (Eds), *Modality and structure in signed and spoken languages* (pp. 422–441). Cambridge: Cambridge University Press. https://doi.org/10.1017/CBO9780511486777.020

Norbury, C. F., Gooch, D., Wray, C., Baird, G., Charman, T., Simonoff, E., … Andrew, P. (2016). The impact of NVIQ on prevalence and clinical presentation of language disorder: Evidence from a population study. *Journal of Child Psychology and Psychiatry* 11, 1247–1257. https://doi.org/10.1111/jcpp.12573

Peppe, S., McCann, J., Gibbon, F. O., Hare, A., & Rutherford, M. (2006). Assessing prosodic and pragmatic ability in children with high functioning autism. *Journal of Pragmatics* 38, 1776–1791. https://doi.org/10.1016/j.pragma.2005.07.004

Petitto, L. A., & Marentette, P. (1991). Babbling in the manual mode: Evidence for the ontogeny of language. *Science* 251(5000), 1483–1496. https://doi.org/10.1126/science.2006424

Pinker, S. (1994). *The language instinct.* New York, NY: William Morrow and Company. https://doi.org/10.1037/e412952005-009

Poizner, H., & Kegl, J. (1992). The neural basis of language and motor behavior: Evidence from American Sign Language. *Aphasiology* 6, 219–256. https://doi.org/10.1080/02687039208248595

Poizner, H., Klima, E. S., & Bellugi, U. (1987). *What the hands reveal about the brain.* Cambridge, MA: The MIT Press.

Quinto-Pozos, D., Forber-Pratt, A., & Singleton, J. L. (2011). Do developmental communication disorders exist in the signed modality? Perspectives from professionals. *Language, Speech and Hearing Services in Schools* 42, 423–443. https://doi.org/10.1044/0161-1461(2011/10-0071)

Quinto-Pozos, D., Singleton, J., & Hauser, P. (2017). A case of Specific Language Impairment in a native deaf signer of American Sign Language. *Journal of Deaf Studies and Deaf Education* 22, 204–218. https://doi.org/10.1093/deafed/enw074

Quinto-Pozos, D., Singleton, J., Hauser, P., Levine, S., Garberoglio, C. L., & Hou, L. (2013). Atypical signed language development: A case study of challenges with visual-spatial processing. *Cognitive Neuropsychology* 30, 332–359. https://doi.org/10.1080/02643294.2013.863756

Roberts, C., & Hindley, P. (1999). Practitioner review: the assessment and treatment of deaf children with psychiatric disorders. *Journal of Child Psychology and Psychiatry* 40, 151–167. https://doi.org/10.1111/1469-7610.00430

Rosenhall, U., Nordin, V., Sandstrom, M., Ahlsen, G., & Gillberg, C. (1999). Autism and hearing loss. *Journal of Autism and Developmental Disorders* 29, 349–357. https://doi.org/10.1023/A:1023022709710

Roy, P., & Chiat, S. (2013). Teasing apart disadvantage from disorder: The case of poor language. In C. R. Marshall (Ed.), *Current issues in developmental disorders* (pp. 125–150). London: Psychology Press.

Shield, A. (2010). *Phonological errors in the sign language of children with autism* (Unpublished doctoral dissertation). University of Texas.

Sieratzki, J. S., Calvert, G. A., Brammer, M., David, A., & Woll, B. (2001). Accessibility of spoken, written, and sign language in Landau-Kleffner syndrome: A linguistic and functional MRI study. *Epileptic Disorders* 3, 79–89.

Smith, N., Hermelin, B., & Tsimpli, I. (2003). Dissociation of social affect and theory of mind in a case of Asperger syndrome. *UCL Working Papers in Linguistics* 15, 357–377.

Smith, N, Tsimpli, I., Morgan, G., & Woll, B. (2011). *The signs of a savant: Language against the odds*. Cambridge: Cambridge University Press.

Tager-Flusberg, H. (1981). On the nature of linguistic functioning in early infantile autism. *Journal of Autism and Developmental Disorders* 11, 45–46. https://doi.org/10.1007/BF01531340

Tallal, P. (2000). Experimental studies of language learning impairments: From research to remediation. In D. V. M. Bishop & L. B. Leonard (Eds.), *Speech and language impairments in children: Causes, characteristics, intervention and outcome* (pp. 135–155). Hove: Psychology Press.

Tomblin, B., Records, N., Buckwater, P. Zhang, X., Smith, E., & O'Brien, M. (1997). Prevalence of specific language impairment in kindergarten children. *Journal of Speech, Language and Hearing Research* 40, 1245–1260. https://doi.org/10.1044/jslhr.4006.1245

Volker, M., Lopata, A. C., Smith, D. A., & Thomeer, M. L. (2009). Facial encoding of children with high functioning autism spectrum disorders. *Focus on Autism and Other Developmental Disabilities* 24, 195–204. https://doi.org/10.1177/1088357609347325

Wellman, H. M., & Peterson, C. C. (2013). Deafness, thought bubbles, and theory-of-mind development. *Developmental Psychology* 49, 2357–2367. https://doi.org/10.1037/a0032419

Woll, B., & Sieratzki, J. S. (1996). Sign language for children with acquired aphasia. *Journal of Child Neurology* 11, 347–348. https://doi.org/10.1177/088307389601100419

Wray, C., Saunders, N., McGuire, R., Cousins, G., & Norbury, C. F. (2017). Gesture production in language impairment: It's quality not quantity that matters. *Journal of Speech, Language, and Hearing Research* 60, 969–982. https://doi.org/10.1044/2016_JSLHR-L-16-0141

CHAPTER 6

Age of acquisition effects in language development

Diane Lillo-Martin, Neil Smith and Ianthi Tsimpli

The most accessible language for deaf children is generally a sign language, but few children have input in sign languages early in life. Late first-language acquisition of a sign language reveals age of acquisition effects that must be taken into consideration by linguistic theories of acquisition. When deaf children access spoken language through a cochlear implant, age of acquisition effects can again be seen, and the presence or absence of sign language is an important factor in language outcomes. Finally, the development of a sign language as a second language in unique contexts such as that of Christopher, a polyglot savant, can reveal more about the nature of language development and the theories of language structure that must be posited.

1. Introduction

Virtually every child with typical hearing receives accessible linguistic input from birth; indeed, some linguistic information is even available *in utero*, as evidenced from linguistic fine-tuning shown by neonates (e.g., Moon et al., 1993; Partanen et al., 2013). Thus, most research on first language acquisition keeps age-of-exposure as a constant. Nevertheless, researchers have been aware of the possibility of age of acquisition (AoA) effects since at least the 1960's, when Lenneberg (1967) proposed that language acquisition is subject to a *Critical Period*. On Lenneberg's proposal, learning a language after the critical period is over would be a significantly different process from acquisition before its closure.

Lenneberg suggested several types of evidence to support his proposed critical period, including adult second language (L2) learning, and young children's recovery of linguistic function following brain injury. But as for children experiencing variation in the age of first linguistic exposure, Lenneberg had to rely on extreme cases in which many other factors, such as social isolation, are relevant (such as the famous case of Genie; Curtiss et al., 1974).

https://doi.org/10.1075/tilar.25.06lil
© 2020 John Benjamins Publishing Company

In the decades since, it has become apparent that the evidence regarding the critical period hypothesis is much more complex (Mayberry & Kluender, 2018). Studies with adults learning a second language have revealed similarities to first-language acquisition, alongside persistent difficulties which might be attributed to a sensitive period for optimal language development (among many others, see Flege et al., 1999; Johnson & Newport, 1989; Smith, 2002). It has become clear that AoA is but one factor that contributes to linguistic development.

Whether there is a critical period for language acquisition is important for numerous reasons. Some have taken its putative existence as an argument for the existence of an innate language-learning mechanism (e.g., Smith, 2005). However, AoA effects could be related to general neural development and not implicate a domain-specific language acquisition device. The proposal of an innate language learning mechanism does not in itself predict or depend on the existence of critical period effects. Either way, if language learning is substantially a different process at age one compared to age fourteen, theories of language development need to account for this. Practically speaking, knowing the cut-off for a critical period – or more likely, which aspects of language are learned differently at which times – could be an important justification for certain educational approaches, such as those encouraging early bilingualism, and could assist in the design of improved language teaching materials.

With these and other issues in mind, researchers have recently addressed a number of new questions related to possible effects of AoA: questions which are among the many topics that Bencie Woll's work has addressed. In this chapter, we summarize selected aspects of this research, drawing connections to her work and her influence, in acknowledgment of the great contribution that her studies have made. We start with relevant background on the critical period hypothesis and on modality effects in language acquisition in Section 2.

It is not possible to ask about potential effects of differences in the age of first linguistic exposure for hearing children, since input in at least one language is available from birth. However, many children who are born deaf are in exactly this situation: at birth, there is no accessible linguistic input presented to them, since they cannot readily access spoken language and the vast majority of children born deaf have hearing, non-signing parents (Mitchell & Karchmer, 2004 estimate that at most 5% of deaf children in the U.S. are born to signing parents). Even if children have extensive interactions with loving parents, it may take years before accessible input is available.

Given this general context, researchers have used variation in age of language access to address questions about possible effects of the AoA of a first language. We start with the cases in which this late first language is a natural sign language. For many deaf people, following a lack of success in learning a spoken language despite oral training, exposure to a natural sign language commences. How that language develops, where modality effects might be seen, and consequences of linguistic delay on both structure and processing will be the topic of the third section of this chapter.

Over the past few decades, the linguistic environment for deaf children has changed substantially, due to the increasing sophistication and availability of hearing technology, such as hearing aids and especially cochlear implants. Nevertheless, cochlear implants have not eliminated possible linguistic effects of deafness, since even very early-implanted infants experience some delay of linguistic input, and the result of implantation is not natural spoken language acquisition but requires extensive training. There is considerable variability in the linguistic outcomes of children who have received cochlear implants (Bruijnzeel et al., 2016; Niparko et al., 2010), some of which may be related to variation in the age of exposure following activation. Effects of AoA for spoken language development in deaf cochlear implant users will be summarized in the fourth section.

Finally, we look at the unique case of the acquisition of a sign language by a linguistic savant. Christopher shows that even in adulthood, there are aspects of language that he can learn easily. However, the linguistic domains of relative strength and weakness for him reveal potential age effects and effects of the linguistic modality. These factors can interact with age in a way that presents great difficulties for adult learners. These findings will be discussed in the fifth section. We will conclude with some implications and connections to Bencie Woll's influence.

2. Background

2.1 Language domains and critical period effects

The consensus of researchers is that talk of 'a critical period' is too simplistic: there is evidence for more than one critical period, as shown by some of Bencie Woll's work (e.g. Woll & Morgan, 2002, p. 292), where the issue is raised whether "the critical periods for native-like acquisition of signed and spoken languages" are identical; and by some of our own work (Berk & Lillo-Martin, 2012; Smith & Tsimpli, 1995, Smith et al., 2011). There are, moreover, partially overlapping critical periods for syntax and phonology and, we contend, a critical period for the acquisition of the core vocabulary of the lexicon (*near, go, table, moon, out, off*, etc. as opposed to *circumnavigate, economy, esoteric* and so on). If this claim is correct, it suggests that second language vocabulary is partly calqued on the first language's vocabulary, with the result that learners find it difficult to master subtle differences between 'equivalent' (or cognate) lexical items in their first and subsequent languages. For example, speakers of Hindi where the word for 'hand' ([ha:th]) includes the fore-arm and the word for 'foot' ([per]) includes the lower leg, may persist in giving the English translations the same extended meaning despite explicit teaching.

Nonetheless, the domain of the Critical Period is quintessentially syntax, which is also the primary locus of parametric variation (Baker, 2008).[1] However, parametric differences can regulate overarching or more detailed properties of language, referred to as macroparameters and microparameters respectively (Biberauer, 2008; Roberts & Holmberg, 2010). Each macroparameter is associated with a number of microparameters which allow for variation within the same macro-type. For example, the OV/VO distinction and the Verb-Second rule (V2) of Germanic languages are macroparameters associated with microparametric options distinguishing further among head-final, V2 languages (Haider, 2012) and are usually associated with morphological distinctions. From this perspective, macroparameters and their associated microparametric options determine the core components of each language.

In monolingual development, the phenomena which are acquired earliest belong to the core and are narrowly syntactic. In first language acquisition, macroparameters are acquired only slightly earlier than microparameters; in second language acquisition, the distinction between macro- and microparameters is more evident and could be associated with age or Critical Period effects (Tsimpli, 2014). Specifically, late bilinguals seem to have problems with the microparametric properties of the core system rather than the macroparametric ones (Kroffke & Rothweiler, 2006). This is mostly due to the *dissociation* between the development of syntax and morphology in second language grammars which has been argued for on theoretical and empirical grounds (Lardiere, 1998; Schwartz, 2009; Smith & Tsimpli, 1995). Thus, although morphology and syntax develop concurrently in L1 acquisition, adult L2 acquisition may show better syntactic than morphological abilities.

2.2   Modality effects and age effects

For the very small percentage of deaf children who acquire a sign language as a native language by exposure from their signing parents, the overall course of language development can be described as parallel to that observed for children acquiring a spoken language (for an overview see Chen Pichler et al., 2018). This population – like those children developing spoken languages – shows no variation

---

1. The conjecture limits syntactic variation to formal features of functional categories and would not include the kind of Hindi example we mentioned above.

in age of exposure, hence no age-of-acquisition effects. However, this is not to say that there are absolutely no differences between acquiring a sign language and acquiring a spoken language; there are significant differences in the modality of sign and spoken languages which can lead to *modality effects* in acquisition. As we discuss potential age of acquisition effects in this chapter, we will attempt to contrast them with potential modality effects, to better understand how these factors may interact.

The first, most apparent modality effect is that sign languages are produced using the hands, face, and body, and perceived through the eyes, while spoken languages are produced using the vocal tract and perceived primarily through the ears (though visual perception of spoken language is also important; see, e.g., Massaro & Simpson, 1987). Thus, signs are generally described by specifying (at least) their handshape, the location in which the sign is made, and the movement of the sign. In addition, certain facial expressions and head positions are associated with various types of linguistic information, including intonational marking of information/discourse structure, adverbials, and negation. This distinction between signed and spoken words, while a surface difference, is relevant to multiple aspects of native first-language acquisition, and potentially to age-of-acquisition effects.

For example, because the manual articulators develop more quickly than the vocal ones, it is possible for signing children to produce recognizable signs somewhat earlier than the first spoken words are produced. Exactly how much difference there is has been debated, but there is arguably at least a one-to two-month difference in the average age of first signs versus first words (Meier & Newport, 1990). In addition, the form of the early signs may differ from adult forms in ways that are determined by modality (Meier et al., 2008). Children's first signed or spoken words show effects of their still-developing phonology and the articulatory control needed. In spoken languages, this can be realized by replacement of certain (marked) phonemes by others (unmarked), change in the number of syllables produced, consonant cluster reduction, and the like. In sign languages, marked handshapes (such as) may be replaced by unmarked ones (such as); joints proximal to the body (shoulder, elbow) may be used when the target requires joints farther from the body (wrist, knuckles), resulting in signs appearing larger; and the child's production may contain a different number of syllables from the adult target. As these descriptions indicate, similar underlying processes can be implicated in a number of cases, but the differences in spoken and sign language development are still tied to differences in the modality of production.

When sign linguists list the modality-based differences between sign languages and spoken languages, they go beyond the surface fact of hands vs. mouth, because modality differences are indeed deeper (e.g., Meier et al., 2002). A compelling and still not fully understood modality difference has to do with the way that 'signing space' is used. While spoken words are uttered in a sequential stream and signs are also uttered in sequence, the signs add a spatial dimension. It has already been mentioned that a sign's location is part of its necessary description. However, when signs are produced in 'neutral space' in front of the signer, additional distinctions can be made, so that spatial differences correspond to verb argument structure, complex representations of motion or spatial descriptions, contrast, and numerous other functions. Because several of these spatially realized differences have been analysed as involving complex morphology, a number of studies of early and later language development have concentrated on them. We will expand on these areas of potential modality effects as we come to studies for which they are relevant in the following sub-sections.

How, then, can we take potential modality effects into consideration while we look at putative effects of age of acquisition? First, we can keep in mind that surface differences in the production of sign versus speech might be relevant. Second, we can look at phenomena that relate to modality differences, such as the use of space, and ask how learners with varied types of experiences do with these phenomena, in comparison (when possible) to other learners and other phenomena. While there are very few studies that can be used to compare effects of age of first-language acquisition of a sign language to a spoken language, as would be necessary to definitively attribute some effect to modality versus age, we will bring up the modality issue throughout this chapter to keep it in the forefront of our consideration.

3.   Late L1 acquisition of sign languages

When a deaf child is born to hearing parents who do not sign, some time is needed for parents to adjust, decide how they want to communicate with their child, and begin to learn how to implement their decision (Young & Tattersall, 2007). If the parents choose to expose their child to a sign language and learn to sign themselves, it will take time for them to do this, and their early efforts will be quite limited; but once a child is exposed to a natural sign language that input will be immediately accessible. If the parents choose to use speech only (possibly with hearing technology for the child), the child will watch their parents' faces as they speak as infants generally do (Dodd, 1979), but the input they receive will be limited; speech training will begin at some point but there will inevitably be some delay, and in some cases, children will subsequently learn a sign language.

A few studies have looked at the course of sign language development by deaf children once they begin to have delayed exposure to a natural sign language. One such study looked at two unrelated deaf children (called Mei and Cal in the literature) who started attending a residential school for the Deaf in the United States around the age of 5–6 years, having had no accessible linguistic input prior to their enrolment (Berk, 2003). This study followed the children for four years, using repeated longitudinal collection of spontaneous production data, as they interacted with a Deaf native signer who provided their primary input in American Sign Language (ASL).

A number of findings about the course of delayed language development emerged from this study. One point was that the children both went through a two-word stage of the type that very young language learners typically do (Berk & Lillo-Martin, 2012); this observation implies that the two-word stage is a function of linguistic development rather than chronological age per se. A separate study of teenage late learners of ASL found the same thing (Ferjan Ramirez et al., 2013).

Within the domain of morphology, a very interesting contrast was observed in the study of Mei and Cal. Mei and Cal displayed a remarkable asymmetry in their use of signing space, not observed in native signers with input from birth. For some verbs, such as HELP,[2] GIVE, SHOW, and ASK, the way they move in space represents the referents involved in an event described by the verb. This use of space is called verb agreement or person marking in much of the sign language literature (see Lillo-Martin & Meier, 2011). Other verbs, known as spatial or locative agreeing verbs (Padden, 1983), including GO, COME, BRING, and MOVE, indicate not their arguments, but the location(s) of the events they denote.

The two uses of space for person agreement and locative agreement look very similar: both involve movement of a verb sign from one location to another. Both also require the locations in space to be associated with their person or locative referents – either because the referent is actually physically there, or through a linguistic association. However, they function differently in several grammatical ways. For Mei and Cal, the two types of space were learned in different ways: both children were able to use signing space correctly with spatial verbs, and both made many errors with person agreeing verbs. Their errors included some failures to use person agreement where it is required as well as some instances of using the wrong location – somewhat analogous to English-speaking children dropping required inflection ('he run') or supplying the incorrect form ('I runs'). They did not improve in their use of space with person agreeing verbs even over the four years of observation

Difficulties with the use of space have been reported in other studies of late learners as well, including those by Newport (1990) and Emmorey et al. (1995), though these studies did not distinguish between person-agreeing and spatial

---

2. As is common in sign linguistics, we use English glosses written in upper case to represent signs that have an overlapping range of meaning.

verbs. We will come back to this commonality after summarizing other findings from late learners.

Ferjan Ramirez et al. (2013) report on early stages of acquisition of ASL by three deaf late first-language learners (Shawna, Cody and Carlos) whose exposure began during adolescence (around age 14, tested after 12–24 months of exposure). They measured the learners' vocabulary using the ASL version of the MacArthur-Bates Communicative Development Inventory (Anderson & Reilly, 2002), and found that their vocabulary size was larger than the norms for typically-developing native ASL signing children with the same length of exposure. Interestingly, the learners showed evidence of discussing concepts that typical 2-year-old learners do not yet know, like computers, sports, and distant events, such as a volcano eruption they learned about at school. They also found that the mean length of utterance (MLU) of the learners was between 2 and 3, which is comparable to native signers between the ages of 1 and 2 years. In many ways these results are comparable to those found by Berk & Lillo-Martin (2012), indicating that at the early stages of acquisition at least, progression is similar whether the delay is relatively less (5–6 years) or more (14 years).

While the studies just summarized examined the first years following immersion in a sign language, a number of studies have looked at adults with decades of experience using a sign language as their primary language. These studies compare adults who had, long before, experienced their first accessible linguistic input at various ages. While many of them might have been in oral-language-based educational programs before they were exposed to a sign language, their development of spoken language was so limited that they are generally considered to be late learners of a first language.

One study (Newport, 1990) looked at performance on a number of ASL tasks by adults in three groups: native signers, whose exposure began from birth, 'early' signers, whose exposure began around the ages of 4–6 years (note that this is the age of exposure for Mei and Cal), and 'late' signers, whose exposure began only after the age of 12 years (the age of exposure for Shawna, Cody and Carlos). Among the assessments these participants took, one was a test of basic word order, which in ASL is Subject – Verb – Object. All three groups, native, early, and late-exposed participants, scored fairly high on this assessment. However, the groups differed in a series of other tests, with the native signers scoring highest, the early learners scoring significantly lower than the native signers, and the late learners scoring significantly lower than the early signers. These tests looked at various aspects of ASL morphology, including verb agreement, and verbs of motion and location, or classifiers. The contrast between performance on basic word order and complex morphology could be a parallel to the proposed Critical Period distinction between macroparameters and microparameters mentioned in

Section 2.1, although the contrast has not been discussed in these terms and more work would be needed to see whether these categories are appropriate for the sign language phenomena.

ASL classifiers are of some interest because of the persistent challenges they pose for learners. Although there is debate about how best to analyse these structures (see papers in Emmorey, 2003), a general, simplified description is as follows. The handshape, which in non-classifier signs is a meaningless component, is chosen to represent a class of referents, such as upright animate beings, vehicles, or long thin objects. This referent might be the subject, object, or instrument of an event which is conveyed through the movement through space of the hand. In order to use a classifier construction accurately, the signer must choose the appropriate handshape for the referent, and produce the movement in such a way as to convey the movement of an entity (possibly between a source and a goal) along with its path and manner. Native signing children begin to use classifiers at an early age (Slobin et al., 2003), but they do not perform at adult-like levels until they are much older (Schick, 1990, among others). Later learners seem to have particular difficulties with tests of their production or comprehension of classifiers. Both the 'early' group and the 'late' group of non-native signers performed much worse than native signers on such structures (Newport, 1990).

A study of two adolescent late learners by Morford (2003) also bears on this issue. She studied two learners, Maria and Marcus, who were 12–14 years old when they were first immersed in ASL. In their first few years of exposure to ASL, both learners began using classifier constructions, but they made errors in their choice of handshape and/or in the accuracy of the movement. When their comprehension was tested 7 years after exposure, both learners performed quite poorly (around chance) at normal processing levels. However, when the learners were allowed to view stimulus videos multiple times and at slow speeds, their performance increased dramatically. This indicates that at least some of the difficulty experienced by late learners might be related to phonological processing issues.

That phonological processing is a particular challenge for late learners is supported by a number of other studies. Mayberry (2010) and Mayberry and Kluender (2018) review a series of studies that were conducted with adults who had been late learners (generally with acquisition starting in adolescence). These participants are long-time users of ASL, but differences between them and native signers have been shown on tests including narrative shadowing and sentence recall. Strikingly, tests of late second-language learners of ASL (participants who became deaf and learned to sign after having learned a spoken language with normal hearing) show much better performance than late first-language learners, indicating that the possible critical period effects for language learning are much different for first-versus second-language learners. As might be expected, these late learners also showed particular problems with ASL morphology, including verb agreement and classifiers.

In one of the few studies that focus on syntactic knowledge as well as ASL morphology, Boudreault and Mayberry (2006) tested native signers, early learners, and delayed learners using a grammaticality judgment task with sentences of differing levels of complexity, including WH-questions and relative clauses, as well as sentences with verb agreement and classifiers. They found that late learners performed significantly worse than native signers overall. Interestingly, the pattern of responses across different types was similar for the three groups, with all groups performing worst on the relative clause sentences.

Cormier et al. (2012) raised a question about the results presented by Boudreault and Mayberry. Since the participants in their study had been involved in oral educational programs prior to their immersion in ASL, it might have been possible that they had learned some English as a first language, so that their ASL results actually reflect L2 learning. This possibility can be discounted for the studies that test the early stages of acquisition (e.g., Berk & Lillo-Martin, 2012; Morford, 2003; Ferjan Ramirez et al., 2013), since the level of learners' knowledge of a spoken/written language at the time of immersion is virtually nil. To address this possibility, Cormier et al. replicated the Boudreault & Mayberry study with signers of British Sign Language (BSL), but also assessed their English knowledge at the time of testing. In this way, they could factor out English reading level in their analyses of the participants' scores on the BSL grammaticality judgment task.

Cormier et al. (2012) found that their delayed learner group (reported immersion in BSL between 9 and 18 years of age) scored significantly higher on the reading test than the early learner group (BSL exposure beginning between 2 and 8). This suggests that the late learner group had some competence in English as an L1 and learned BSL as an L2. This might relate to the result that only the early learner group (not the late learners) showed a decrease in accuracy on the grammaticality judgment task as their age of first exposure to BSL increased.

The proposal by Cormier et al. (2012) that (at least some) participants who are classified as late L1 learners of a sign language might actually be L2 learners should be considered when evaluating suggestions that learners like Shawna, Cody and Carlos are more severely affected by their late exposure than learners who were in oral educational programs (Mayberry & Kluender, 2018). It is impossible to know without a decades-long longitudinal study, but the possibility remains that the majority of late learners in most research studies have a slight advantage, with at least some aspects of language accessed before their exposure to sign language. The widespread differences between such participants and native signers (or late known L2 signers) indicate, however, that whatever might have been gained before exposure to a sign language did not suffice to serve as equivalent to a full natural first-language, whether signed or spoken.

To sum up, a series of studies have indicated that delayed exposure to language for children born deaf will have profound consequences on language development which persist into adulthood. While the effects are widespread, they are not uniform; there is evidence that some areas of language are more severely affected than others. We have raised the possibility that the distinction between areas more and less severely affected would correspond to the distinction between macroparameters and microparameters that has been proposed to account for differences in L2 acquisition effects. In particular, the relative sparing of word order in simple sentences versus the greater difficulty with more complex syntax (such as ones with relative clauses) is potentially compatible with this division. It remains to be seen whether the distinction between spatial and person agreeing verbs observed by Berk (2003) is – if replicated – also amenable to such an explanation.

4. Deaf children with cochlear implants

The studies reviewed in the previous section demonstrated that delayed exposure to a sign language as a first language can have serious, long-lasting effects on linguistic development and processing. Many deaf children are likely to face such delay while parents learn to sign and/or the child's educational placement provides sign input. But in the past few decades, the options for deaf children have expanded with the introduction of paediatric cochlear implantation and universal new-born hearing screening leading to early identification and intervention (Yoshinaga-Itano, 2009). Does the introduction of a cochlear implant and subsequent spoken language development alleviate the challenges children face in delayed language acquisition?

Although cochlear implants are increasingly recommended at earlier ages, with many children receiving surgery even before 12 months, there is still a time-period during which deaf children cannot readily access spoken language before the implant is inserted and activated (Levine et al., 2016). Much research has observed that even when participants are chosen from those with the greatest likelihood of success with a cochlear implant, results are quite variable. Even for those who received their implants before 18 months of age, three years later the mean of their expressive and receptive language scores was equivalent to hearing children two years younger, with a large variation (Niparko et al., 2010). While it is clear that results are better for those implanted in the first few years, what accounts for the range of results even within the early-implant group?

Some researchers have argued that exposure to a visual language before im-plantation and/or during rehabilitation contributes to lower levels of success (e.g. Geers et al., 2017). There have been a number of studies that compare spoken lan-guage outcomes in deaf children who have received CIs and then been educated using oral only approaches vs. those who have had some amount of sign language and/or visual linguistic input (e.g., cued speech). The results are mixed; some show equivalent outcomes (e.g., Jiménez et al., 2009), others show an advantage for oral only (e.g., Peterson et al., 2010). However, these studies almost never measure the quality or quantity of the visual language input or the child's development of sign; they simply group together all children who have had any amount of visual input (Caselli et al., 2017). What are the findings if children's sign proficiency is also considered?

In a very few studies, the children's proficiency in sign language is measured or can be assumed. Hassanzadeh (2012) and Davidson et al. (2014) tested spoken language outcomes in deaf children from deaf, signing families, after the children had received cochlear implants. Both studies found that these participants showed much better spoken language development (in Persian, Hassanzadeh; or in English, Davidson et al.) in comparison to non-signing deaf CI users. Davidson et al. fur-thermore found that the native signers showed (chronological) age-appropriate scores on standardized tests, which were not distinct from the scores of hearing children of deaf parents.

Despite the suggestive results from native signers, some researchers have maintained that exposure to sign language is deleterious for spoken language development in cochlear-implanted children (e.g., Geers et al., 2017). They argue that visual linguistic input leads to take-over of auditory neural areas, which subsequent auditory input through the implant cannot override. Two papers from Woll and her colleagues review the evidence and make a strong case against this conclusion (Lyness et al., 2013; Campbell et al., 2014).

First, it is important to point out two observations about neural areas for language processing: (a) brain areas used for sign language largely overlap with those used for spoken language; (b) spoken language processing itself is multi-modal, with a significant role of vision. Neural areas for language are known to be multi-modal (or amodal) (see also Cardin et al., Chapter 9 of this volume). As for the primary auditory areas, Lyness et al. (2013) and Campbell et al. (2014) review studies that have purported to find dystrophic processing due to visual stimulation, and conclude that there is no convincing evidence for such an effect. Campbell et al. (2014, p. 8) conclude that disordered cortical circuitry which has been observed is "more likely to be associated with disordered language learning in the sensitive early years," since auditory deprivation and language deprivation are typically confounded. Lyness et al. (2013) suggest that when children do receive accessible visual language input in the early period, normal development of amodal brain areas for language will take place, and that this is crucial for brain readiness for spoken language after implantation.

The conclusion by Campbell et al. (2014) and Lyness et al. (2013) is that differences in how the brain processes language between deaf CI users and hearing non-signers are more likely to be due to delayed linguistic exposure in the former and not specifically their lack of auditory input or their exposure to visual language input. Since the age of implantation is now increasingly younger, such a result indicates that some critical period(s) close off at a very early age, even if some language development is still achieved by learners with exposure at early school age or even adolescence. What properties of language crucially require input in the first year of life?

The most likely conclusion is that the optimal period to begin language exposure is right after birth, because important perceptual processes for both spoken language and sign language develop during this time (e.g., Werker & Tees, 1984; Stone et al., 2017). As Morford and Mayberry (2000) have argued, phonological development typically takes place in this first year, and delays or disruptions in this development will have cascading effects in other linguistic domains. The longer accessible input is delayed, the more profound these effects are.

So far, we have seen clear evidence for effects of the age of acquisition of a sign language for those born deaf, for whom spoken language development cannot take place in the typical way. What kinds of effects might be found in those children or adults who are learning a sign language as a second language? While there is relatively less research in this area, one point that is clear is that modality effects must be taken into consideration, since most learners of a sign language as L2 are also learning a language in a new modality, or M2 (Chen Picher, 2012; Chen Pichler & Koulidobrova, 2015). To what extent do M2L2 learners transfer linguistic knowledge from their L1, as spoken language L2 learners frequently do? Do M2L2 learners show Critical Period effects such as those discussed in Section 2.1, distinguishing between macroparameters and microparameters? It is not possible to answer such questions for typical adult M2L2 learners here, but they can be addressed from the point of view of an atypical learner: Christopher, a linguistic savant who learned BSL.

5. Sign language acquisition in an atypical case: What Christopher can tell us

Christopher, born in January 1962, is an individual who has been institutionalized all his adult life because he is unable to look after himself. His case demonstrates an asymmetrical pattern between cognition and language with the latter spared in comparison with the former. On standardized measures of non-verbal cognition he scores between 40 and 75, while his verbal abilities are within the upper range of the scale (O'Connor & Hermelin, 1991; Smith & Tsimpli, 1995; and references therein).

Christopher's profile becomes unique when one turns to language. Apart from English, his native language, Christopher speaks and/or understands twenty other languages to different degrees. His language learning abilities exhibit an extremely fast and accurate pattern mostly for languages which have a written form, although his ability to learn signed languages lacking written feedback, while weaker overall, still reveals a special talent for language compared to non-verbal abilities (Smith et al., 2011).

An in-depth investigation of his linguistic abilities reveals further asymmetries *within* his languages. Starting with English, Christopher's mastery of morphology and vocabulary are intact, but his syntactic abilities show a diverse pattern. For instance, although subordination, in the form of relative and adverbial clauses, interrogatives and parasitic gaps, is clearly part of Christopher's native grammar, topicalisation and left-dislocation are not. He does not use these constructions himself and rejects examples of them produced by others as ungrammatical. Other aspects of his language performance are also affected in apparently different ways. For instance, Christopher's translations into English (from a variety of languages) occasionally fail to meet criteria of coherence and pragmatic plausibility; interpreting non-literal language can also be distressing. Smith et al. (2011) have interpreted these findings as reflecting a demarcation between structures which reflect higher and lower discourse-sensitivity. The contrast is then between the intact status of 'formal' aspects of Christopher's English on the one hand, and discourse-related structures which are affected for independent reasons, such as his communication deficit, on the other. Christopher's performance on comparable discourse-sensitive structures in his other L2s (e.g. Greek, French, Spanish) is also problematic, presumably for similar pragmatic reasons (Smith & Tsimpli, 1995).

BSL also fits this overall picture: Christopher's mastery of the formal side of BSL – the morphology and syntax – is superior to his use of BSL for communication. Christopher's performance on BSL becomes more impressive when one considers his severe apraxia, his limited visuo-spatial, kinaesthetic and social abilities. BSL was the first signed language he was exposed to, and as he was explicitly instructed in BSL (rather late considering the other languages he learned), it was clearly a 'foreign' language to him. Nevertheless, Christopher's learning of BSL was within the same range of achievement as that of a comparison group of university undergraduates given the same syllabus.

In order to address possible critical period effects in Christopher's acquisition of second languages we can exclude pragmatically-relevant syntactic structures, as these require the integration of macroparametric and microparametric properties with discourse-related information, external to the language core. We can thus directly compare Christopher's mastery of formal properties of his L1 with those of his L2s, signed and spoken. As both BSL and all of his 'second' spoken languages were taught either in adolescence or in adulthood they qualify as 'late' L2s, i.e. languages acquired post-critical period. Apart from L1 vs. L2 syntax, we can also focus on similarities and differences in morphology and the lexicon of Christopher's BSL and spoken languages to identify candidate areas for critical period effects.

The evidence: Christopher's signed and spoken languages

A dissociation between syntax and morphology has been attested in second language grammars. Christopher's language learning in general also shows such a dissociation, although his profile goes the opposite way: he excels at morphology (however complex – e.g. he coped easily and enthusiastically with the morphology of Berber), and at the lexicon (his vocabulary in 20 languages is remarkable) while his L2 syntax rapidly reaches a plateau beyond which he is unable to progress. In all, Christopher's spoken L2s diverge from the average L2 learner who, with exposure, is expected to perceive, accept and eventually produce structures that do not exist in the L1. Christopher's L2 syntax was different from his English L1 mostly in cases when L2 morphology – which was easily mastered – allowed him to infer syntactic properties. In this respect, we can suggest that critical period effects are responsible for blocking some aspects of L2 syntactic development which in the typical L2 learner may be circumvented by employing compensatory linguistic or cognitive mechanisms (Smith & Tsimpli, 1995; Hawkins & Hattori, 2006; Tsimpli & Dimitrakopoulou, 2007).

The situation becomes more complex when we turn to the signed modality. Despite his (mild) autism and consequent reluctance to make eye contact, Christopher learned BSL to a standard comparable with a comparison group of talented second language learners in comprehension tasks (comprehension is the appropriate measure since production was compromised by his severe apraxia). Apart from being taught and tested on the lexicon of BSL, Christopher and the comparison group were exposed to negative and interrogative sentences, subject and object agreement verbs and classifiers encoding spatial relations.

The main asymmetry observed in Christopher's performance was between classifier predicates, a structure in which most of the comparison group performed very well, and the other syntactic structures in which he was similar to the other participants, albeit at the lower end of the range. Notably, Christopher showed minimal transfer effects from English on BSL sign order in interrogative, declarative and negative sentences, a remarkable difference from all of his other spoken languages for which English word order is his preferred choice. Despite the fact that his BSL production was very limited, Christopher exhibited good progress in developing knowledge of the BSL syntax of negation, less so in verbs encoding subject and object agreement such as GIVE, ASK, LOOK, HELP, TEACH, etc., and most poorly in classifier predicates encoding spatial relations. His inability to process and judge spatial information with classifier predicates stands in contrast with the performance of deaf late language learners and of the hearing learners of BSL included in the comparison group of the study.

We have proposed that the gradual decline in Christopher's performance in the three structures (negation, agreement, classifiers) could be explained by comparing the contribution of spatial processing to linguistic processing in each case (Smith et al., 2011, p. 167). Given Christopher's deficit in visuo-spatial processing, it is inevitable that higher demands on linguistic processing would accrue in classifier structures encoding spatial relations followed by subject-and-object agreement predicates. If our analysis is correct, then the signed modality affected Christopher's development of BSL morpho-syntax in specific structures, something that we had not observed in his spoken languages even when the linguistic representation encoded spatial relations. The lack of a written form of BSL input also deprived him of the opportunity to detect morphological information and develop the same level of morphological awareness he appears to have in his spoken L2s. Modality effects were also found in Christopher's performance on the BSL lexicon where iconicity did not seem to facilitate his recognition of signs as it did in many participants of the comparison group (Smith et al., 2011, p. 186).

Overall, Christopher's learning of BSL revealed three areas where modality seemed to affect performance positively or negatively. Positive effects of the signed modality were found in the absence of negative transfer effects from English on the sign order in his BSL sentences. While it is not clear what it is about the modality of sign languages that should lead to such an effect, the fact that this pattern was distinct from his performance on all spoken languages leads us to consider it a modality effect. An unexpected absence of modality effects was attested in the acquisition of the sign lexicon where iconicity did not seem to improve his performance, unlike what we found in every member of the comparison group. Finally, negative effects of the signed modality were found in the acquisition of classifier predicates where Christopher clearly struggled, unlike the other BSL learners, but like the late L1 learners of ASL discussed in Section 3.

Christopher is not like a typical L2 learner either in his spoken or signed languages. His profile is better than the average L2 learner's in the very fast and accurate development of the L2 lexicon and morphology and worse in that core syntactic structures seem to stagnate. The overpowering influence of his English L1 on his spoken languages indicates that not just complex syntax but also main parametric properties of the macro- and micro-type are problematic for Christopher. Whether this is an indication of a selective critical period effect on L2 acquisition remains an open question.

6. Conclusions and implications

We have reported several domains in which effects of the age of acquisition of a language can be observed, and a hypothesis about how critical periods for language dissociate different linguistic components. Further work is needed to test the hypothesized distinctions more thoroughly, particularly in the context of sign language acquisition (as late L1 or M2L2). In particular, late L1 learners may have a broader range of effects, which are more pronounced the longer the period of language deprivation extends. Which properties can still be learned for late L1 learners (core vocabulary, simple syntax?), and how they relate to common difficulties for L2 and M2L2 learners will be a persistent area of research (cf. Mayberry & Kluender, 2018). Furthermore, the observation that difficulties in spatial aspects of BSL might be related to more general visual-spatial problems for Christopher leads to the possibility that similar difficulties in late L1 learners call for testing of general visual-spatial abilities.

Special circumstances of language learning allow for extensive testing of theoretical proposals about critical periods, something that continues to be of great interest. We see Bencie Woll's contributions to critical period research as promoting such theoretical questions, but more importantly, she also stressed the practical issue of language access for deaf children. In this domain, we fully agree with the conclusions that Campbell et al. (2014, p. 8) come to:

> good first language acquisition within the early years, however that may be achieved, may be the best predictor of successful language outcome for the child born deaf.

References

Anderson, D., & Reilly, J. (2002). The MacArthur communicative development inventory: Normative data for American Sign Language. *Journal of Deaf Studies and Deaf Education* 7(2), 83–106. https://doi.org/10.1093/deafed/7.2.83

Baker, M. (2008). The macroparameter in a microparametric world. In T. Biberauer (Ed.), *The limits of syntactic variation* (pp. 351–373). Amsterdam: John Benjamins. https://doi.org/10.1075/la.132.16bak

Berk, S. (2003). *Sensitive period effects on the acquisition of language: A study of language development* (Unpublished doctoral dissertation). University of Connecticut, Storrs.

Berk, S., & Lillo-Martin, D. (2012). The two-word stage: Motivated by linguistic or cognitive constraints? *Cognitive Psychology* 65, 118–140. https://doi.org/10.1016/j.cogpsych.2012.02.002

Biberauer, T. (2008). Doubling vs. omission: Insights from Afrikaans negation. In S. Barbiers, O. Koeneman, M. Lekakou, & M. van der Ham (Eds.), *Microvariations in syntactic doubling* (pp. 103–140). Bingley: Emerald.

Boudreault, P., & Mayberry, R. (2006). Grammatical processing in American Sign Language: Age of first-language acquisition effects in relation to syntactic structure. *Language and Cognitive Processes* 21(5), 608–635. https://doi.org/10.1080/01690960500139363

Bruijnzeel, H., Ziylan, F., Stegeman, I., Topsakal, V., & Grolman, W. (2016). A systematic review to define the speech and language benefit of early (<12 months) pediatric cochlear implantation. *Audiology and Neurotology* 21, 113–126. https://doi.org/10.1159/000443363

Campbell, R., MacSweeney, M. & Woll, B. (2014). Cochlear implantation (CI) for prelingual deafness: The relevance of studies of brain organization and the role of first language acquisition in considering outcome success. *Frontiers in Human Neuroscience, 8,* Article 834. https://doi.org/10.3389/fnhum.2014.00834

Caselli, N., Hall, W. & Lillo-Martin, D. (2017). Operationalization and measurement of sign language. (Commentary on paper by Ann Geers et al.) *Pediatrics* 140(5), e20172655B. https://doi.org/10.1542/peds.2017-2655B

Chen Pichler, D. (2012). Language acquisition. In R. Pfau, B. Woll & M. Steinbach (Eds.), *Sign language: An international handbook* (pp. 647–686). Berlin: De Gruyter. https://doi.org/10.1515/9783110261325.647

Chen Pichler, D., & Koulidobrova, E. (2015). Acquisition of sign language as a second language. In M. Marschark (Ed.), *The Oxford handbook of deaf studies in language: Research, policy and practice* (pp. 218–230). Oxford: Oxford University Press.

Chen Pichler, D., Kuntze, M., Lillo-Martin, D., de Quadros, R. M., & Stumpf, M. (2018). *Sign language acquisition by deaf and hearing children: A bilingual introduction.* Washington, DC: Gallaudet University Press.

Cormier, K., Schembri, A., Vinson, D., & Orfanidou, E. (2012). First language acquisition differs from second language acquisition in prelingually deaf signers: Evidence from sensitivity to grammaticality judgement in British Sign Language. *Cognition* 124, 50–65. https://doi.org/10.1016/j.cognition.2012.04.003

Curtiss, S., Fromkin, V., Krashen, S., Rigler, D., & Rigler, M. (1974). The linguistic development of Genie. *Language* 50(3): 528–554. https://doi.org/10.2307/412222

Davidson, K., Lillo-Martin, D., & Chen Pichler, D. (2014). Spoken English language development among native signing children with cochlear implants. *Journal of Deaf Studies and Deaf Education* 19(2), 238–250. https://doi.org/10.1093/deafed/ent045

Dodd, B. (1979). Lip reading in infants: Attention to speech presented in-and out-of-synchrony. *Cognitive Psychology* 11, 478–484. https://doi.org/10.1016/0010-0285(79)90021-5

Emmorey, K. (Ed.). (2003). *Perspectives on classifier constructions in sign languages*. Mahwah, NJ: Lawrence Erlbaum Associates. https://doi.org/10.4324/9781410607447

Emmorey, K., Bellugi, U., Friederici, A. & Horn, P. (1995). Effects of age of acquisition on grammatical sensitivity: Evidence from on-line and off-line tasks. *Applied Psycholinguistics* 16(1), 1–23. https://doi.org/10.1017/S0142716400006391

Ferjan Ramirez, N., Lieberman, A., & Mayberry, R. (2013). The initial stages of first-language acquisition begun in adolescence: When late looks early. *Journal of Child Language* 40(2), 391–414. https://doi.org/10.1017/S0305000911000535

Flege, J., Yeni-Komshian, G., & Liu, S. (1999). Age constraints on second-language acquisition. *Journal of Memory and Language* 41, 78–104. https://doi.org/10.1006/jmla.1999.2638

Geers, A., Mitchell, C., Warner-Czyz, A., Wang, N., & Eisenberg, L. (2017). Early sign language exposure and cochlear implantation benefits. *Pediatrics* 140, 1–9. https://doi.org/10.1542/peds.2016-3489

Haider, H. (2012). *Symmetry breaking in syntax*. Cambridge: Cambridge University Press. https://doi.org/10.1017/CBO9781139084635

Hassanzadeh, S. (2012). Outcomes of cochlear implantation in deaf children of deaf parents: Comparative study. *The Journal of Laryngology & Otology* 126(10), 989–994. https://doi.org/10.1017/S0022215112001909

Hawkins, R., & Hattori, H. (2006). Interpretation of English multiple wh-questions by Japanese speakers: A missing uninterpretable feature account. *Second Language Research* 22, 269–301. https://doi.org/10.1191/0267658306sr269oa

Jiménez, M., Pino, M., & Herruzo, J. (2009). A comparative study of speech development between deaf children with cochlear implants who have been educated with spoken or spoken+sign language. *International Journal of Pediatric Otorhinolaryngology* 73, 109–114. https://doi.org/10.1016/j.ijporl.2008.10.007

Johnson, J., & Newport, E. (1989). Critical period effects in second language learning: The influence of maturational state on the acquisition of English as a second language. *Cognitive Psychology* 21(1), 60–99. https://doi.org/10.1016/0010-0285(89)90003-0

Kroffke, S., & Rothweiler, M. (2006). Variation im frühen Zweitspracherwerb des Deutschen durch Kinder mit türkischer Erstsprache. In M. Vliegen (Ed.), *Proceedings of the 39th Linguistics Colloquium* (pp. 145–153). Bern: Peter Lang.

Lardiere, D. (1998). Dissociating syntax from morphology in a divergent L2 end-state grammar. *Second Language Research* 14, 359–375. https://doi.org/10.1191/026765898672500216

Lenneberg, E. (1967). *Biological foundations of language*. New York, NY: John Wiley and Sons. https://doi.org/10.1080/21548331.1967.11707799

Levine, D., Strother-Garcia, K., Golinkoff, R., & Hirsh-Pasek, K. (2016). Language development in the first year of life: What deaf children might be missing before Cochlear implantation. *Otology & Neurotology* 37(2), e56–e62. https://doi.org/10.1097/MAO.0000000000000908

Lillo-Martin, D., & Meier, R. (2011). On the linguistic status of 'agreement' in sign languages. *Theoretical Linguistics* 37, 95–141. https://doi.org/10.1515/thli.2011.009

Lyness, C., Woll, B., Campbell, R., & Cardin, V. (2013). How does visual language affect cross-modal plasticity and cochlear implant success? *Neurosci. Biobehav. Rev.* 37, 2621–2630. https://doi.org/10.1016/j.neubiorev.2013.08.011

Massaro, D., & Simpson, J. (1987). *Speech perception by ear and eye: A paradigm for psychological inquiry.* Hove: Psychology Press.

Mayberry, R. (2010). Early language acquisition and adult language ability: What sign language reveals about the critical period for language. In M. Marschark & P. Spencer (Eds.), *Oxford handbook of deaf studies, language and education* (Vol. 2; pp. 281–290). New York, NY: Oxford University Press.

Mayberry, R., & Kluender, R. (2018). Rethinking the critical period for language: New insights into an old question from American Sign Language. *Bilingualism: Language and Cognition* 21, 886–905.

Meier, R., & Newport, E. (1990). Out of the hands of babes: On a possible sign advantage in language acquisition. *Language* 66,1–23. https://doi.org/10.1353/lan.1990.0007

Meier, R., Cormier, K., & Quinto-Pozos, D. (Eds.). (2002). *Modality and structure in signed language and spoken language.* Cambridge: Cambridge University Press. https://doi.org/10.1017/CBO9780511486777

Meier, R., Mauk, C., Cheek, A., & Moreland, C. (2008). The form of children's early signs: Iconic or motoric determinants? *Language Learning and Development* 4, 393–405. https://doi.org/10.1080/15475440701377618

Mitchell, R., & Karchmer, M. (2004). Chasing the mythical ten percent: Parental hearing status of deaf and hard of hearing students in the United States. *Sign Language Studies* 4(2), 138–163. https://doi.org/10.1353/sls.2004.0005

Moon, C., Cooper, R., & Fifer, W. (1993). Two-day-olds prefer their native language. *Infant Behav. Dev.* 16, 495–500. https://doi.org/10.1016/0163-6383(93)80007-U

Morford, J. (2003). Grammatical development in adolescent first-language learners. *Linguistics* 41(4), 681–721. https://doi.org/10.1515/ling.2003.022

Morford, J., & Mayberry, R. (2000). A reexamination of "Early Exposure" and its implications for language acquisition by eye. In C. Chamberlain, J. Morford, & R. Mayberry (Eds.), *Language acquisition by eye* (pp. 111–128). Mahwah, NJ: Lawrence Erlbaum Associates.

Newport, E. (1990). Maturational constraints on language learning. *Cognitive Science* 14(1): 11–28. https://doi.org/10.1207/s15516709cog1401_2

Niparko, J., Tobey, E., Thal, D., Eisenberg, L., Wang, N.-Y., Quittner, A., & Fink, N. (2010). Spoken language development in children following cochlear implantation. *JAMA: Journal of the American Medical Association* 303(15), 1498–1506. https://doi.org/10.1001/jama.2010.451

O'Connor, N., & Hermelin, B. (1991). A specific linguistic ability. *American Journal on Mental Retardation* 95, 673–680.

Padden, C. (1983). *Interaction of morphology and syntax in American Sign Language* (Unpublished doctoral dissertation). University of California, San Diego.

Partanen, E., Kujala, T., Näätänen, R., Liitola, A., Sambeth, A., & Huotilainen, M. (2013). Learning-induced neural plasticity of speech processing before birth. *PNAS* 110, 15145–15150. https://doi.org/10.1073/pnas.1302159110

Peterson, N., Pisoni, D., & Miyamoto, R. (2010). Cochlear implants and spoken language processing abilities: Review and assessment of the literature. *Restorative Neurology and Neuroscience* 28, 237–250.

Roberts, I., & Holmberg, A. (2010). Introduction. In T. Biberauer, A. Holmberg, I. Roberts, & M. Sheehan (Eds.), *Parametric variation: Null subjects in minimalist theory* (pp. 1–56). Cambridge: Cambridge University Press.

Schick, B. (1990). The effects of morphosyntactic structure on the acquisition of classifier predicates in ASL. In C. Lucas (Ed.), *Sign language research: Theoretical issues* (pp. 358–374). Washington, DC: Gallaudet University Press.

Schwartz, B. (2009). Unraveling inflection in child L2 development. *Acquisition et Interaction en Langue Étrangère* 1(1), 63–88.

Slobin, D. I., Hoiting, N., Kuntze, M., Lindert, R., Weinberg, A., Pyers, J., et al. (2003). A cognitive/functional perspective on the acquisition of "classifiers". In K. Emmorey (Ed.), *Perspectives on classifier constructions in sign languages* (pp. 271–296). Mahwah, NJ: Lawrence Erlbaum Associates.

Smith, N. (2002). Jackdaws, sex and language acquisition. In *Language, bananas and bonobos: Linguistic problems, puzzles and polemics*. Oxford: Blackwell.

Smith, N. (2005). Backlash. In *Language, frogs and savants: More linguistic problems, puzzles and polemics*. Oxford: Blackwell.   https://doi.org/10.1002/9780470775059.ch9

Smith, N., & Tsimpli, I. (1995). *The mind of a savant: Language-learning and modularity*. Oxford: Basil Blackwell.

Smith, N., Tsimpli, I., Morgan, G., & Woll, B. (2011). *The signs of a savant: Language against the odds*. Cambridge: Cambridge University Press.

Stone, A., Petitto, L.-A., & Bosworth, R. (2017). Visual sonority modulates infants' attraction to sign language. *Language Learning and Development* 14, 130–148. https://doi.org/10.1080/15475441.2017.1404468

Tsimpli, I. (2014). Early, late or very late? Timing acquisition and bilingualism. *Linguistic Approaches to Bilingualism* 4(3), 283–313.   https://doi.org/10.1075/lab.4.3.01tsi

Tsimpli, I., & Dimitrakopoulou, M. (2007). The interpretability hypothesis: Evidence from *Wh*-interrogatives in L2 acquisition. *Second Language Research* 23, 215–242. https://doi.org/10.1177/0267658307076546

Werker, J., & Tees, R. (1984). Cross-language speech perception: Evidence for perceptual reorganization during the first year of life. *Infant Behavior and Development* 7(1), 49–63. https://doi.org/10.1016/S0163-6383(84)80022-3

Woll, B., & Morgan, G. (2002). Conclusions and directions for future research. In G. Morgan & B. Woll (Eds.), *Directions in sign language acquisition* (pp. 291–299). Amsterdam: John Benjamins.   https://doi.org/10.1075/tilar.2.15wol

Yoshinaga-Itano, C. (2009). Universal newborn hearing screening programs and developmental outcomes. *Audiological Medicine* 1, 199–206.   https://doi.org/10.1080/16513860310002031

Young, A., & Tattersall, H. (2007). Universal newborn hearing screening and early identification of deafness: Parents' responses to knowing early and their expectations of child communication development. *Journal of Deaf Studies and Deaf Education* 12, 209–220. https://doi.org/10.1093/deafed/enl033

CHAPTER 7

Links between language and cognitive development of deaf children

Gary Morgan, Anna Jones and Nicola Botting

This chapter weaves together work on early interaction between parents and children who are deaf or hard of hearing (DHH) with research on social-emotional development (Theory of Mind) and wider cognitive abilities (Executive Functions). We describe in detail why language input in sign or spoken language (or both together) facilitates the development of communication, language and cognitive skills using what has been termed the Language Scaffolding Hypothesis. The chapter concludes with a discussion of what research is required next to understand how the current language learning experiences of DHH children – the majority who will have a cochlear implant and hearing parents – can promote both language and cognitive development.

1.   Introduction

Language develops in children so they can understand others, as well as to express themselves fully. It is one of the most important abilities for all children to master as it links up with cognition, aiding children to solve problems, remember and make plans. Children use language to ask their first questions, make their first friends, as well as recount their first stories and learn about the world around them. There are many pieces involved in enabling children to learn language without seemingly being explicitly taught how to do it. The social-interaction piece of the story is that language development grows out of innumerable instances of parents, carers and siblings interacting with the young child. In these interactions the acquisition of words or signs is not the primary aim of the interlocutors; rather, they are focused on successful interpersonal communication and intersubjectivity (Trevarthen & Hubley, 1978; Bruner, 1983; Tomasello, 2008).

   In this framework, the goal of interactions between the infant and the adult is reciprocation through turn-taking games like 'I do something then you respond to it' (Stern & Gibbon, 1979). Infants and their caregivers are sensitive to signals

https://doi.org/10.1075/tilar.25.07mor

to communicate (Tomasello, 1988). Successful communication acts as a scaffold for later acquisition of language. Once children are using words and beginning to form sentences we can say that they are communicating more effectively with a shared language. The child's growth of language facilitates a shared communication about objects and concepts. Infants who share attention with adults and understand intentions when they are hearing language can start to enter into the ensuing stage of learning about what labels that are more abstract refer to, and can also start thinking about the world more generally (Tomasello, 2008). This way of describing early communication development is characterised as a coming together of social-emotional and cognitive systems. This coming together develops out of interaction and thus provides the foundation stones for doing higher-level cognition – for example, thinking about others or planning a sequence of actions. This framework for thinking about language development as happening through interaction puts more emphasis on why infants would require language in the first place rather than the product of that development.

A child who experiences an early disruption with communication because of difficulties with interaction and poor exposure to language can be at two disadvantages. First, this situation can lead to delays in social-emotional development due to early difficulties with interaction and joint attention (Vaccari & Marschark, 1997; see Harris and Clibbens chapter on early interaction in this volume). Secondly, poor exposure to language can cause major difficulties with the structural aspects of spoken and/or sign language because of audiological access and poor input factors. This chapter reviews the current literature on delays in spoken and sign language development in deaf and hard of hearing (DHH) children next, before exploring the potential consequences of these delays for wider cognitive abilities.

2.   What is the impact of deafness on language development?

Around 5–10% of DHH children are born to deaf parents (DCDPs). These children typically learn a sign language, which is generally the native or primary language of their parents. As such, deaf children in this situation receive native-like language input since the parents communicate more or less effortlessly with their children in fully functional language. Research has described the acquisition of sign language in DCDPs as resembling that of typically-developing hearing children with respect to the onset, rate, and pattern of early language development (Morgan & Woll, 2002; Schick, Marschark, & Spencer, 2005), although as yet we do not know enough about later stages of sign language development. For this group of deaf children, then, there is relatively little impact of their deafness on their language development.

The other 90–95% of DHH children have hearing parents (DCHP, Mitchell & Karchmer, 2004). Many of these children learn a spoken language, while others learn a sign language. Each of these paths presents difficulties for language development. Spoken language development in children born congenitally deaf is increasingly facilitated by cochlear implantation (CI), which is rapidly becoming the norm in Europe and North America as an audiological intervention for DCHPs. CIs are typically offered to children in these regions following a neo-natal diagnosis of deafness. At present the age of CI is decreasing, and in some countries is as low as 12 months or younger (see Levine et al., 2016, for an overview of why age of implantion is important). Across many studies of spoken language development in DHH children, however, one common theme is that there is great variability in outcomes (Geers, Nicholas, Tobey, & Davidson, 2016). The possible impact of this on the language system is explored in the previous chapter on critical periods (Lillo-Martin, Tsimpli, & Smith, this volume).

It is important to note that CIs do not instantly turn a DHH child into a hearing child with typically developing language. One main reason for this is the lack of language input between birth and the time when the CI begins functioning effectively. Between diagnosis and implantation, DHH children will be fitted with hearing aids and so experience variable sound stimulation. However, the age of implantation can often be up to 24 months and in some cases as late as 36 months. Thus, the important early period for the development of phonology and early word learning, the establishment of communication through interaction, and the development of intersubjectivity can be compromised. Despite an early CI there are periods of months at a time where the CI teams are programming and mapping the CI to the child's environment and during this time sounds and linguistic input will not be fully accessible leading to delays in the onset of spoken language development.

Another group of DHH children typically learn a signed language. For many, this is because they are not candidates for a CI because of medical or physical characteristics such as a non-functional auditory nerve. For others, the initial use of a CI does not lead to successful spoken language development and so families turn to a sign language as their only alternative. Still other children are in families who choose to use a sign language rather than a CI from the outset, though these situations are becoming relatively rare. Importantly in all these situations, the exposure to a sign language for DCHPs typically comes from their hearing parents who are rarely native speakers of this language, and most did not use a sign language before the birth of the child. In other words, the children's primary language input, especially at young ages, tends to be from non-native speakers with limited proficiency in the language.

Learning any second language as an adult is labour intensive and for hearing parents, who need to learn to sign while their child is very young, the parents are learning to communicate with their child during the most sensitive period for language exposure (see chapter by Cardin et al., this volume, and Schick, Marschark, & Spencer, 2005). There is not only a time pressure, but also most sign language instruction does not focus on child-directed language. This inevitably means that many DCHP are first exposed to a low quality sign input. Further, this sign input often only begins after the first few years of development (Lu et al., 2016) and in a decreasing number of children during early teens (Morford, 2002). Thus, for the DCHP who might be more reliant on a sign language for communication, there is challenge for them to acquire the language because of a lack of necessary fluent models. In addition, it is probably the case that hearing parents learn sign vocabulary and use this in conjunction with speech rather than full-blown signed language grammar. It has not been investigated in enough detail what constitutes 'language' input spread across both modalities for a DCHP.

Hearing children do not only learn language in the home but instead are exposed to many sources of input around them. This situation is different for DCHP, who if exposed to sign input might only see a single adult signing. If this is so, these children will inevitably miss out on incidental learning from exposure to language around them. It is unlikely, for example, that two hearing parents will sign with each other if not directly including their deaf child, at least in the first years of learning the language.

Crucially, we know very little about the real content of early input in situations where DCHP have a sign language as their primary language, and there are numerous questions about what constitutes sign input to a DCHP overall. In contrast, we know much more about the quality and quantity of the early oral input to DCHP who have a spoken language as their primary language (see next section for details), perhaps because DCHP with spoken input typically receive extensive speech and language therapy and there is a large research base on this topic,

We can summarise the previous information as the impact of deafness on development is variable. DHH children exposed to a signed language from their deaf parents establish typical levels of interaction leading to joint attention, intersubjectivity and subsequently language development. DCHP are in a potentially at risk situation of language delays because of the possible disruptions to early social interaction and attainment of intersubjectivity. Coupled with this are two reduced language learning situations where in the first 12 months deafness is a barrier for full access to spoken language and parent's initially can only provide poor models of sign language. We can look at longer term influences of early difficulties in communication on two major aspects of cognitive development: theory of mind and executive functions.

3. Language for cognitive development: Theory of Mind and Executive Functions

Theory of Mind (ToM) is the human social-cognitive ability to connect with one another at the level of inner and unobservable mental states such as knowledge and beliefs. The development of children's ToM has been a major research topic for the last 30 years. Recently, attention has turned to the environmental enablers of social cognition found in early parent–child interaction. Several studies included DHH children's performance on ToM experiments (understanding of False Belief) in an attempt to ask if full language development is necessary for development of social cognition.

In the early studies, all kinds of children labelled 'deaf' were grouped together because, at that time, it was thought that the simple fact of being deaf prevented a child from developing a full-blown ToM. Across these children there was a wide variability in early experience with language and interaction (Spencer & Meadow-Orlans, 1996). Further, the inclusion of both DCHP and DCDP children in one group meant that the role of the early communicative environment (Peterson, 2004; Siegal & Surian, 2011) and language development (Schick, de Villiers, de Villiers, & Hoffmeister, 2007) in promoting ToM were conflated. All of these factors led to substantial difficulty in interpreting the results of the early ToM studies with deaf children. Eventually, two main studies were conducted using large sample sizes of DCDPs, with typical language development and no social or cognitive impairments. Both studies found no ToM delays compared to hearing peers. This demonstrated that, rather than deafness per se leading to delays, early experience of good interaction and language exposure in deaf children led to typical ToM development (UK: Woolfe, Want, & Siegal, 2002 and USA: Schick, de Villiers, de Villiers, & Hoffmeister, 2007). These studies therefore reignited questions about why variability in early interaction experienced by DCHPs would lead to ToM delays. The UK group pursued the argument that early participation in conversation was a vital element in ToM development, while the American group favoured the development of syntactic skills.

This coincided with a shift in how ToM development was being described more generally. Wellman and Lui (2004) made the point that earlier research which posited a 'radical conceptual shift' between 4–5 years of age – the age at which children start to pass False Belief tasks – was underestimating children's ToM abilities. Wellman and Lui (2004) proposed a continuum or scale of ToM abilities beginning during the first year. At this age infants begin to demonstrate joint attention understanding and are beginning to grasp the internal intentions of others (Tomasello, Carpenter, Call, Behne, & Moll, 2005); both these skills provide an essential foundation for more complex ToM reasoning abilities. The scale proposes progression from simple to more complex mental state understanding with one part of this progression being the understanding of false beliefs. How these early sensitivities develop or trigger later higher-level ToM is still being debated and the study of DHH children has provided useful indications. Because early abilities in understanding others might be linked to the quality of the interaction children experience, DCHP can shed light on how early disruptions and difficulties in establishing joint attention and inter-subjectivity can have later consequences. This research fits into the social-interaction framework outlined at the outset of the chapter and revisits quite early research which described various aspects of the early communicative experiences of DCHP (Lederberg & Mobley, 1990; Wedell-Monnig & Lumley, 1980). It also provides some evidence for why some DHH children might have difficulty with ToM.

During their first year of life, typically hearing infants take part in countless interactions with their parents. Interaction using shared language in these contexts is a way of gaining the attention of the infant – for monitoring and commenting on the infant´s actions and for guiding the attention of the infant to outer and inner experiences (Meins, Fernyhough, Arnott, Leekam, & de Rosnay, 2013; Morgan, Meristo, & Hjelmquist, 2014). A number of studies highlight the importance of both the presence of mental state labels in the caregiver input and the type of conversation style. These interactions provide ToM-triggering content (language) as well as high quality social-interaction. For example, in studies of hearing children by Meins et al. (2013), parents´ references to mental states of their infant at 6 months of age were predictive of ToM at four years of age. Morgan, Meristo, Mann, Hjelmquist, & Siegal, (2014) carried out an analysis of conversational experiences of DHH and hearing children aged 17–35 months, all with hearing parents. The majority of the children knew spoken and signed language although language levels varied greatly. Parents were asked to describe pictures that elicited mental and emotional state language to their children. The input to the DCHP from parents differed greatly in terms of mental state labels compared with hearing parents talking to their hearing same-age children. Parents of hearing children referred to cognition (i.e., using words like 'think', 'know' or 'remember') significantly more often than did those of DCHP children. There were no differences between groups in references to desires or emotions. These findings support the argument that early conversations influence the development of ToM understanding. Parents might tune their ToM-related language to the language level of the child rather than the older chronological age (Fagan, Bergeson, & Morris, 2014).

The quality of social interaction is a second important factor that forms the foundation for later ToM abilities. In addition to the reduced or simplified content of interactions, many studies have demonstrated differences in the quality of social interaction in families with DHH children. Recall that the Wellman & Lui (2004) scale includes early interaction as a pre-requisite for more complex ToM developments. It is these types of early interactions, which are affected by childhood deafness. Studies of the interaction style of hearing mothers of DHH children compared to hearing mothers of hearing children described the former group as demonstrating a more directive style that resulted in less participation and initiation from the children. The authors argued that this adaptation meant the DHH children were less able to interpret their mothers' intentions (Lederberg & Mobley, 1990).

Another part of this framework is the idea that contingency between inter-locutors or the connectedness of a conversation is important for ToM (Astington & Baird, 2005). Connected talk overlaps with feelings of closeness with your conversation partner. Early research refers to mothers' anxiety and feelings of in-competence in how to interact with a DHH child and this has been suggested as a possible cause for interruptions in maternal responsiveness (Spencer & Meadow-Orlans, 1996). There are also differences in how the timing of interactions changes when the child is DHH versus hearing. Spencer, Bodner-Johnson and Gutfreund (1992) reported that deaf mothers were much more likely to wait for their child to look back at them before responding than hearing mothers of DHH children (70% of time compared to only 16% of time by hearing mothers). Morgan et al. (2014) found that the hearing-parent/hearing-child dyads produced significantly more connected turns than the hearing-parent/deaf-child dyads. Parents with a DHH child thus have difficulty maintaining a conversation and are less likely to immediately relate their language directly to the infants' previous turn.

Several studies of DHH children of hearing parents have reported delays in establishing and using joint attention with their parents (see Harris & Clibbens, this volume). In contrast, when DHH children are immersed in an environment with sufficient visual communication with deaf parents, they develop joint attention skills at the same age and follow the same stages as hearing children (Harris & Clibbens, this volume; Nowakowski, Tasker, & Schmidt, 2009). DCDP spend just as much time in coordinated joint attention as hearing-parent/hearing-child pairs at 18 months, but DCHP spend a reduced total amount of time in joint attention at this age (Lieberman, Hatrak, & Mayberry, 2014).

A number of studies have looked at responsiveness linked to joint attention in greater detail. Deaf mothers of deaf children are reported to be more respon-sive to changes in attention marked by their children's small shifts in eye gaze. Hearing mothers were more likely to miss these subtle signals or misinterpret them as inattention from the deaf child (Swisher, 1992). For the deaf mother, their child making eye-contact is interpreted as a request and looking away is a new topic initiation or an opportunity for their child to scan their environment before returning their gaze (Kyle, Woll, & Ackerman, 1989; Loots, Devisé, & Jacquet, 2005; see chapter by Harris & Clibbens, this volume).

In summary, evidence suggests that DCHP have a different quality of early interactional experience in terms of more directive input, less mental state content of conversations, less maternal responsiveness and less joint attention and contingency. This reduced quality of experience might provide fewer triggers for the development of early intersubjectivity and the range of ToM related abilities that grow during this time. This delay should be distinguished from ToM impairments demonstrated by children with Autism. DCHP follow the same progression on the ToM scale from simple to more complex mental state understanding as do hearing children but this progression is considerably delayed (Peterson, Wellman, & Slaughter, 2012). Importantly, when studies include a language-age control group (younger hearing children), the gap between hearing and DHH children on ToM tasks reduces, but it is still significantly wider than would be expected (e.g. Netten et al., 2015). This reinforces the argument that language helps ToM development but on its own is insufficient. It is early communicative experiences that lead to eventual language-mediated ToM skills. This last point reinforces the idea that interventions should not focus solely on speech and language but rather use of language in interaction.

A second area of cognitive development which builds on early experience of language is Executive Functions (EF). EFs are a set of abilities which enable us to coordinate mental processes and manipulate information, solve novel problems, sequence information, and generate new strategies to accomplish goals in a flexible way (Elliott, 2003; Funahashi, 2001). The relationship over development between EF and language is a major interest for researchers and clinicians in hearing children with typical and atypical development. This is because there is a growing realisation that children with variable skills in language might also struggle with EF. There has been a small number of studies yielding data on this topic in DHH children (e.g. Figueras, Edwards, & Langdon, 2008) including two large studies by our own group (Botting et al., 2017; Jones et al., 2019).

There are three possible theoretical explanations for a developmental link between language and EF (e.g., Fuhs & Day, 2011; Kuhn et al., 2014). First, language skills may enhance EF via the ability to use vocabulary as labels to create internal representations (as described in the Cognitive Complexity and Control [CCC] theory: Zelazo & Frye, 1998). Second, EF might support language acquisition by increasing selective attention and enabling the child to monitor several sources of information at the same time in order to make decisions (Diamond, 2013; Weiland, Barata, & Yoshikawa, 2014). Third, the relationship may be reciprocal, and language and EF may influence one another in development (Bohlmann, Maier, & Palacios, 2015).

Given that EF and language might influence each other, it has been difficult to untangle the direction of influence from previous research with hearing children who receive full language input from birth. This is different to the language deficits seen in DCHP which typically reflect delayed rather than disordered functioning.

In the wider literature, there is a position that draws quite stark conclusions on the impact of deafness on EF development and is reminiscent of the idea discussed in the previous section of this chapter on ToM. Previously in the chapter, we described this position: deafness in itself (i.e., audiological deprivation) precluded a child developing a full-blown ToM. The same position has been proposed for EFs, based on the notion that speech perception/exposure is the crucial factor in predicting EF. From this work, the 'Auditory Scaffolding Hypothesis' emerged (Conway, Pisoni, & Kronenberger, 2009).

However, the inclusion of DCDP with early exposure to accessible communication in some of the samples of the EF studies has revealed that for this group at least, DHH children can display age-appropriate EFs (Marshall et al., 2015; Hall, Eigsti, Bortfeld, & Lillo-Martin, 2017). In terms of language affecting EF, typical development of EFs in DHH children is again conditional on the child having had an early experience of language and communication – in other words, having deaf parents who provide accessible and fluent language input. It might well be the case that DCHP who are exposed to degraded sound-based language and poor levels of signing have difficulties with auditory scaffolding of cognition. Without the protective factors of good early interactions, these difficulties could persist into later childhood. It is not clear at this time how much language (signed, spoken, or both) is enough to facilitate the development of a functioning EF system. There are two parts to this question: how much language and how early does this need to be present for the young child (see Pierce, Genesee, Delcenserie, & Morgan, 2017, for a recent review of this question).

The Cardin, et al chapter in this volume explores the effects on brain plasticity because of auditory deprivation on the one hand, and exposure to language early or late in development on the other. The evidence suggests that DCDP have intact and age appropriate EF skills (Marshall et al., 2015; Hall, Eigsti, Bortfeld, & Lillo-Martin, 2017). However, these two studies were limited in that the first looked only at non-verbal working memory and the second used a parent measurement of child EF – the BRIEF – rather than assessing EF directly in the child. In summary, having early high quality language input from deaf parents may well protect the young DHH child from EF delays. However, early access to high quality language is an exception if you are a DHH child, since some 95% of DHH children have hearing parents. We do not know that if hearing parents could communicate to the same level in sign language as deaf parents do whether this would lead to EF and indeed ToM developing appropriately. In addition, spoken language communication is difficult to establish for a section of the young CI population. Thus, EF delays need to be explained within the wider DCHP population.

In contrast to the Auditory Scaffolding Hypothesis is the Language Scaffolding Hypothesis. In Botting et al. (2017) and Jones et al. (2019), we posited a strong direction of influence from language to EF development. We also nuanced this hypothesis by suggesting that there were two routes to EF development stemming from early language development: one from the interaction afforded by a shared fully accessible language system (inter-subjectivity again), and the second based on the power of language to support inner speech and problems solving. The small number of studies exploring language and EF in DHH children have reached different conclusions. Remine, Care and Brown (2008) found no association between language and EF, while Figueras et al. (2008) found that while DHH had lower EF and language scores than same-age hearing comparisons, EF and language were highly associated. In two recent studies from our group (Botting et al., 2017 and Jones et al., 2019) we looked at this question with a large sample of DHH and hearing children (aged 6–11 years) across two time points (24 months apart). Both DHH and hearing children were assessed on language and several nonverbal EF tasks. Botting et al. (2017) report that even though the DHH sample presented with no cognitive disorder, the DHH children as a group scored below their hearing peers on the majority of EF tasks. The finding that DHH children's EF task performance was significantly lower remained even after accounting for speed of processing and nonverbal ability, and despite the tasks being carefully chosen for their nonverbal demands. We carried out an analysis of all the children's vocabulary skills (which we used as a proxy for language) and found that while language mediated group differences in EF skill, the reverse pattern was not evident. In a follow-up paper (Jones et al., 2019), we reported on a sub-section of DHH and hearing children from Botting et al. (2017) tested on EF and language two years later. Findings were positive in that all children improved their scores on all tasks over this period, but the DHH children performed significantly less well than hearing peers on some EF tasks and on the vocabulary test. Regression models showed that vocabulary at Time 1 predicted change in EF scores for both DHH and hearing children, but not the reverse (Jones et al, 2019).

As described in several chapters in this volume, the DHH population is extremely heterogeneous in terms of language and cognitive abilities. In order to test the language-EF link, it is important not only to have DCDP in the sample but also data on the other factors thought to influence language and cognitive skills. These factors include whether children use a CI or a hearing aid, length of CI and hearing-aid use, age of onset of hearing aid use and/or implantation, type of educational setting, and level of competence on a range of non-verbal abilities. It is also important to have children with a range of language skills. This last factor is worth describing in more detail. Prior to starting the Botting et al. (2017) study, we assembled an advisory panel of researchers (deaf and hearing) and those who work clinically or in deaf education (for example, teachers and speech and language therapists). One of the recommendations made by the then head of the British Association of Teachers of the Deaf was to recruit a sample that came from mainstream schools rather than from specialist deaf schools. The rationale was that this was the most representative type of educational setting that DHH children were in at the time (indeed there are now even larger numbers of DHH children in mainstream schooling than at this earlier period). When we collected language and cognitive data in mainstream schools, we were confronted by a sample that in the majority used spoken language rather than signed language.

While this preference for spoken language had increased, it did not mean that the language was age appropriate. In Jones et al. (2016), we described in detail the spoken language skills of the DHH sample in our EF study. In agreement with many previous studies, it was found that the DHH group had poorer control of English grammatical morphemes as well as reference forms (he, she, it, etc.), and that this added to their lower expressive vocabulary skills. Thus, we concluded from this work that even though DHH children were making gains in terms of spoken language development (possibly as a result of early identification of deafness, widespread inclusion in mainstream schooling, and increased speech perception), language development delay was still an issue. This meant that language and EF were poorer in DHH children than in their hearing peers, and we argued that these two factors were related. Our current position is that both EF and language grow out of early communicative experiences that children experience in the first years of life, and that this relationship is developmentally vulnerable.

As outlined briefly previously, there are two possibilities why disruption to early intersubjectivity and language development might lead to difficulties in the efficient use of EFs: (1) the role of interaction and regulation and (2) the role of private speech/sign. Firstly, several researchers have highlighted the important role of maternal interaction as important for vocabulary development but also as a promoter of emotional and cognitive regulation (Lowe et al., 2012; Hughes, White, & Ensor, 2014). Hearing children and probably DCDP are surrounded by adults who use language to regulate and foster self-regulation through scaffolding of communication.

Secondly, better language skills would also mean a more fully developed use of private speech or sign. During several higher level cognitive tasks such as those requiring EFs (planning, working memory, and inhibition), a language-delayed DHH child is less likely to be able to exploit private speech. Lidstone, Meins, and Fernyhough (2012) found that 7- to 11-year-old hearing children with language impairments used less optimal private speech, on the EF task Tower of London.

We are unsure if DHH children with poor language development use private speech or sign. In the Vygotskian (1962) model, private speech develops from early social interaction and we know that DCHPs experience disruptions in this area (e.g., Fagan et al., 2014). A study of private speech/sign in language delayed DHH children with environmental causes, provides a theoretically useful comparison with hearing children who have language impairments stemming from a cognitive-neurological deficit.

The opening framework of this chapter highlighted the importance of social interaction for language development. It is possible, as described for ToM development, that good early interactions may promote both private speech and lexical development necessary for EF skills. Deafness can lead to delays in the establishment of early EF skills, as well as the later implementation of language resources to assist EFs through private speech. Indeed, these two elements may be more or less present depending on the particular EF task. For example, working memory, inhibition and fluency might be more sensitive to early developmental disruptions (Best & Miller, 2010). However, a planning EF task may be more reliant on concurrent implementation of private speech and language labels, in line with the CCC framework. The role of private speech in DHH children for problems with EF has not been investigated to date, despite some support that vocabulary score mediates EF performance in this group (Botting et al., 2017; Jones et al., 2019; Marshall et al., 2015).

4.   General conclusions

The study of DHH children highlights how early interaction is crucial for language development and related cognitive abilities. DCDP demonstrate appropriate early language and cognitive development possibly because their parents are familiar and experienced in effectively communicating with their child in the language that the child can most easily access. DCHP would benefit from this rich linguistic environment, but the question is how can those effective strategies used by deaf parents be made feasible and accessible to hearing parents? There is a pressing need to create and systematically evaluate early interventions aimed at increasing communication abilities that have a positive consequence for language skills. If language development can be achieved via excellent communication, research suggests this will foster age appropriate cognitive abilities. However, the key problem is that it remains a challenge for DCHP to experience early access to communication through high-level sign language communication with their hearing parents. If parents are using spoken language there are a number of challenges to perceiving all the necessary input, as well as the adaptations hearing parents make to the quality of the conversational environment. A future set of research projects are needed around the variability observed in language outcomes following CI. Two main factors underling this variation in outcome are the quality of communication/language of hearing parents (across the speech-sign spectrum) and the ability of future CIs to increase access to spoken language interventions. Future work based on this research can impact on how DHH children are supported in the family and early school settings. Thus early speech/sign language and communication interventions should have a major component on communication, interaction and inter-subjectivity, as well as a CI and spoken language therapy. As Bencie Woll has said many times, the visual and spoken aspects of languages need not compete with each other but if either is neglected there can be long-lasting effects on full cognitive development (Woll, 2018).

This chapter has reviewed the literature on two important areas of cognitive development for DHH children – Theory of Mind and Executive Functions – both of which are reliant on high-level interaction and language. The Language Scaffolding Hypothesis unites how both these cognitive domains develop from early language. Achieving a workable solution to improving the quality of early interaction and language development therefore has the potential to make a significant impact on DHH children's wider development.

References

Astington, J. W., & Baird, J. (2005). *Why language matters for Theory of Mind*. Oxford: Oxford University Press.   https://doi.org/10.1093/acprof:oso/9780195159912.001.0001

Best, J. R., & Miller, P. H. (2010). A developmental perspective on executive function. *Child Development* 81(6), 1641–1660.   https://doi.org/10.1111/j.1467-8624.2010.01499.x

Bohlmann, N. L., Maier, M. F., & Palacios, N. (2015). Bidirectionality in self-regulation and expressive vocabulary: Comparisons between monolingual and dual language learners in preschool. *Child Development* 86(4), 109.   https://doi.org/10.1111/cdev.12375

Botting, N., Jones, A., Marshall, C., Denmark, T., Atkinson, J., & Morgan, G. (2017). Nonverbal executive function is mediated by language: A study of deaf and hearing children. *Child development* 88(5), 1689–1700.   https://doi.org/10.1111/cdev.12659

Bruner, J. S. (1983). *Child's talk: Learning to use language*. New York, NY: Norton.

Conway, C, M,, Pisoni, D. B., & Kronenberger, W. G. (2009). The importance of sound for cognitive sequencing abilities the auditory scaffolding hypothesis. *Current Directions in Psychological Science* 18(5), 275–279.   https://doi.org/10.1111/j.1467-8721.2009.01651.x

Diamond, A. (2013). Executive functions. *Annual Review of Psychology* 64, 135–168.   https://doi.org/10.1146/annurev-psych-113011-143750

Elliott, R. (2003). Executive functions and their disorders imaging in clinical neuroscience. *British Medical Bulletin* 65, 49–59.   https://doi.org/10.1093/bmb/65.1.49

Fagan, M. K., Bergeson, T. R., & Morris, K. J. (2014). Synchrony, complexity and directiveness in mothers' interactions with infants pre- and post-cochlear implantation. *Infant Behavior & Development* 37(3), 249–257. https://doi.org/10.1016/j.infbeh.2014.04.001

Figueras, B., Edwards, L., & Langdon, D. (2008). Executive function and language in deaf children. *Journal of Deaf Studies and Deaf Education* 13(3), 362–377. https://doi.org/10.1093/deafed/enm067

Fuhs, M. W., & Day, J. D. (2011). Verbal ability and executive functioning development in preschoolers at head start. *Developmental Psychology* 47(2), 404–416. https://doi.org/10.1037/a0021065

Funahashi, S. (2001). Neuronal mechanisms of executive control by the prefrontal cortex. *Neuroscience Research* 39, 147–165. https://doi.org/10.1016/S0168-0102(00)00224-8

Geers, A. E., Nicholas, J. G., Tobey, E., & Davidson, L. (2016). Persistent language delay versus late language emergence in children with early cochlear implantation. *Journal of Speech, Language and Hearing Research* 59(1), 155–170. https://doi.org/10.1044/2015_JSLHR-H-14-0173

Hall, M., Eigsti, I., Bortfeld, H., & Lillo-Martin, D. (2017). Auditory deprivation does not impair executive function, but language deprivation might: Evidence from a parent-report measure in deaf native signing children. *The Journal of Deaf Studies and Deaf Education* 22, 9–21. https://doi.org/10.1093/deafed/enw054

Hughes, C., White, N., & Ensor, R. (2014). How does talk about thoughts, desires, and feelings foster children's socio-cognitive development? Mediators, moderators and implications for intervention. In K. H. Lagattuta (Ed), *Children and emotion. New insights into developmental affective sciences* (pp. 95–105). Basel: Karger.

Jones, A., Marshall, C., Botting, N., Atkinson, J., Toscana, E., Denmark, T., Herman, R., & Morgan, G. (2016). Narrative skills in deaf children who use spoken English: dissociations between macro and microstructural devices. *Research in Developmental Disabilities* 59, 268–282. https://doi.org/10.1016/j.ridd.2016.09.010

Jones, A., Atkinson, J., Marshall, C., Botting, N., St Clair, M. C., Morgan, G. (2019). Expressive vocabulary predicts non-verbal executive function: A 2-year longitudinal study of deaf and hearing children. *Child Development*. https://doi.org/10.1111/cdev.13226

Kuhn, L. J., Willoughby, M. T., Wilbourn, M. P., Vernon-Feagans, L., & Blair, C. B. (2014). Early communicative gestures prospectively predict language development and executive function in early childhood. *Child Development* 85, 1898–1914. https://doi.org/10.1111/cdev.12249

Kyle, J. G., Woll, B., & Ackerman, J. A. (1989). *Gesture to sign and speech*. Bristol: Centre for Deaf Studies.

Lederberg, A., & Mobley, C. (1990). The effect of hearing impairment on the quality of attachment and mother–toddler interaction. *Child Development* 61, 1596–1604. https://doi.org/10.2307/1130767

Levine, D., Strother-Garcia, K., Hirsh-Pasek, K., & Golinkoff, R. M. (2016). Language development in the first year of life: What deaf children might be missing before cochlear implantation. *Otology & Neurotology* 37, 56–62. https://doi.org/10.1097/MAO.0000000000000908

Lidstone, J., Meins, E., & Fernyhough, C. (2012). Verbal mediation of cognition in children with specific language impairment. *Development and Psychopathology* 24(2), 651–660. https://doi.org/10.1017/S0954579412000223

Lieberman, A. M., Hatrak, M., & Mayberry, R. (2014). Learning to Look for Language: Development of joint attention in young deaf children. *Language Learning and Development* 10, 19–35. https://doi.org/10.1080/15475441.2012.760381

Loots, G., Devisé, I., & Jacquet, W. (2005). The impact of visual communication on the intersubjective development of early parent–child interaction with 18- to 24-month-old deaf toddlers. *Journal of Deaf Studies and Deaf Education* 10, 357–375. https://doi.org/10.1093/deafed/eni036

Lowe, J. R., MacLean, P. C., Duncan, A. F., Aragón, C., Schrader, R. M., Caprihan, A., & Phillips, J. P. (2012). Association of maternal interaction with emotional regulation in 4 and 9 month infants during the still face paradigm. *Infant Behavior & Development* 35(2), 295–302. https://doi.org/10.1016/j.infbeh.2011.12.002

Lu, J., Jones, A. & Morgan, G. (2016). The impact of input quality on early sign development in native and non-native language learners. *Journal of Child Language* 43, 537–552. https://doi.org/10.1017/S0305000915000835

Marshall C., Jones A., Denmark T., Mason K., Atkinson J., Botting N., & Morgan G. (2015). Deaf children's non-verbal working memory is impacted by their language experience. *Front. Psychol* 6, 527. https://doi.org/10.3389/fpsyg.2015.00527

Meins, E., Fernyhough, C., Arnott, B., Leekam, S., & de Rosnay, M. (2013). Mind- mindedness and Theory of Mind: Mediating roles of language and perspectival symbolic play. *Child Development* 84(5): 1777–1790. https://doi.org/10.1111/cdev.12061

Mitchell, R., & Karchmer, M. (2004). When parents are deaf versus hard of hearing: Patterns of sign use and school placement of deaf and hard-of-hearing children. *The Journal of Deaf Studies and Deaf Education* 9, 133–152. https://doi.org/10.1093/deafed/enh017

Morford, J. P. (2002). Why does exposure to language matter? In T. Givón & B. Malle (Eds.), *The evolution of language from pre-language* (pp. 329–341). Amsterdam: John Benjamins. https://doi.org/10.1075/tsl.53.18mor

Morgan, G., & Woll, B. (Eds.). (2002). *Directions in sign language acquisition*. Amsterdam: John Benjamins. https://doi.org/10.1075/tilar.2

Morgan, G., Meristo, M., & Hjelmquist, E. (2014). Conversational experience, language and the development of Theory of Mind. In V. Slaughter (Ed.), *Environmental influences on Theory of Mind development: Festschrift for Candi Peterson*. Hove: Psychology Press.

Morgan, G., Meristo, M. Mann, W., Hjelmquist, E., Surian, L., & Siegal, M. (2014). Mental state language and quality of conversational experience in deaf and hearing children. *Cognitive Development* 29, 41–49. https://doi.org/10.1016/j.cogdev.2013.10.002

Netten, A. P., Rieffe, C., Theunissen, S., Soede, W., Dirks, E., & Briaire, J. (2015). Low empathy in deaf and hard of hearing (pre) adolescents compared to normal hearing controls. *PLoS ONE* 10(4): e0124102. https://doi.org/10.1371/journal.pone.0124102

Nowakowski, M. E., Tasker, S. L., & Schmidt L. A. (2009). Establishment of joint attention in dyads involving hearing mothers of deaf and hearing children, and its relation to adaptive social behavior. *American Annals of the Deaf* 154(1),15–29. https://doi.org/10.1353/aad.0.0071

Pierce, L., Genesee, F., Delcenserie, A., & Morgan, G. (2017). Variations in phonological working memory: Linking early language experiences and language learning outcomes. *Applied Psycholinguistics* 38(6), 1265–1300. https://doi.org/10.1017/S0142716417000236

Peterson, C. C. (2004). Theory of Mind development in oral deaf children with cochlear implants or conventional hearing aids. *Journal of Child Psychology and Psychiatry* 45, 1096–1106. https://doi.org/10.1111/j.1469-7610.2004.t01-1-00302.x

Peterson, C. C., Wellman, H. M., & Slaughter, V. (2012). The mind behind the message: Advancing theory of mind scales for typically developing children, and those with deafness, autism, or Asperger Syndrome. *Child Development* 83, 469–485.

Remine, M. D., Care, E., & Brown, P. M. (2008). Language ability and verbal and nonverbal executive functioning in deaf students communicating in spoken English. *Journal of Deaf Studies and Deaf Education* 13, 531–545.   https://doi.org/10.1093/deafed/enn010

Schick, B., Marschark, M., & Spencer, P. (Eds.). (2005). *Advances in the sign language development of deaf and hard-of-hearing children*. New York, NY: Oxford University Press. https://doi.org/10.1093/acprof:oso/9780195180947.001.0001

Schick, B., de Villiers, P., de Villiers, J., & Hoffmeister, R. (2007). Language and theory of mind: A study of deaf children. *Child Development* 78, 376–396. https://doi.org/10.1111/j.1467-8624.2007.01004.x

Siegal, M., & Surian, L. (2011). *Access to language and cognitive development*. Oxford: Oxford University Press.   https://doi.org/10.1093/acprof:oso/9780199592722.001.0001

Spencer, P., Bodner-Johnson, B., & Gutfreund, M. (1992). Interacting with infants with a hearing loss: What can we learn from mothers who are deaf? *Journal of Early Intervention* 16, 64–78.   https://doi.org/10.1177/105381519201600106

Spencer, P., & Meadow-Orlans, K. (1996). Play, language, and maternal responsiveness: A longitudinal study of deaf and hearing infants. *Child Development* 67, 3176–3191. https://doi.org/10.2307/1131773

Stern, D. N., & Gibbon, J. (1979). Temporal expectancies of social behaviors in mother–infant play. In A. W. Siegman & S. Feldstein (Eds.), *Of speech and time. Temporal speech patterns in interpersonal contexts*. Hillsdale, NJ: Lawrence Erlbaum Associates.

Swisher, M. V. (1992). The role of parents in developing visual turn-taking in their young deaf children. *American Annals of the Deaf* 137, 92–100.   https://doi.org/10.1353/aad.2012.1086.

Tomasello, M (1988) The role of joint attentional processes in early language development. *Language Sciences* 10, 69–88.   https://doi.org/10.1016/0388-0001(88)90006-X

Tomasello, M. (2008). *Origins of human communication*. Cambridge, MA: The MIT Press.

Tomasello, M., Carpenter, M., Call, J., Behne, T., & Moll, H. (2005). Understanding and sharing intentions: The origins of cultural cognition. *Behavioral and Brain Sciences* 28(5), 675–691. https://doi.org/10.1017/S0140525X05000129

Trevarthen, C., & Hubley, P. (1978). Secondary intersubjectivity: Confidence, confiding and acts of meaning in the first year. In A. Lock (Ed.), Action, gesture and symbol: The emergence of language (pp. 183–229). New York, NY: Academic Press.

Vaccari, S. & Marschark, M. (1997). Communication between parents and deaf children: Implications for social-emotional development. *Journal of Child Psychology and Psychiatry* 38, 793–801.   https://doi.org/10.1111/j.1469-7610.1997.tb01597.x

Vygotsky, L. S. (1962). The problem and the approach. In *Thought and language* (pp. 1–11). Cambridge, MA: The MIT Press.   https://doi.org/10.1037/11193-001

Wedell-Monning, J., & Lumley, J. M. (1980). Child deafness and mother–child interaction. *Child Development* 51, 766–774.   https://doi.org/10.2307/1129463

Weiland, C., Barata, M., & Yoshikawa, H. (2014). The co-occurring development of executive function skills and receptive vocabulary in preschool-aged children: A look at the direction of the developmental pathways. *Infant and Child Development* 23(1), 4–21. https://doi.org/10.1002/icd.1829

Wellman, H. M., & Liu, D. (2004). Scaling of theory of mind tasks. *Child Development* 75, 523–541.   https://doi.org/10.1111/j.1467-8624.2004.00691.x

Woll, B. (2018). The consequences of very late exposure to BSL as an L1. *Bilingualism: Language and Cognition*, 1–2. https://doi.org/10.1017/S1366728918000238

Woolfe, T., Want, S. C., & Siegal, M. (2002). Signposts to development: Theory of Mind in deaf children. *Child Development* 73, 768–778. https://doi.org/10.1111/1467-8624.00437

Zelazo, P. D., & Frye, D. (1998). Cognitive complexity and control, II: The development of executive function in childhood. *Current Directions in Psychological Science* 7(4), 121–126. jstor.org/stable/20182520

CHAPTER 8

Perception and production of language in the visual modality

Implications for sign language development

Matthew W. G. Dye and Robin L. Thompson

Sign language acquisition requires learning how to comprehend and produce a linguistic system that is visual in nature, as opposed to spoken language acquisition which uses the auditory-visual modality. In this chapter, we consider the impact this has for a child acquiring a sign language. We summarize the research literature on sign language production and comprehension, and attempt to integrate psycholinguistic studies with work documenting the visual perceptual abilities of deaf children. While much of this research emphasizes the experience-dependent nature of language processing abilities, reinforcing the importance of early exposure for native-like acquisition, we caution against overgeneralizing from studies of adult processing and call for more child-specific language studies related to comprehension and production within varying acquisition environments.

Since the seminal work of Stokoe, Klima and Bellugi, and others, sign language research has come a long way. No longer is there a concern to demonstrate that these visual-gestural communication systems are natural languages – that is now widely accepted (see Emmorey, 2000, and Sandler & Lillo-Martin, 2006, for overview). Instead, more recent research has attempted to document and understand how sign languages differ from spoken languages, in order to inform our understanding of what language is (Meier, Cormier, & Quinto-Pozos, 2002; Schlenker, 2018) and how it shapes thought (Emmorey, 2002; Marschark, Siple, Lillo-Martin, Campbell, & Everhart, 1997), learning (Marschark & Hauser, 2008), and social interaction (Kyle & Woll, 1985). In this chapter, we focus on our understanding of the comprehension and production of sign languages and what the implications are for sign language acquisition. Language comprehension and production are psychological processes that permit us to understand others' utterances, and to formulate utterances of our own that can be understood, respectively. We will start with comprehension and review research on the visual perception of sign

https://doi.org/10.1075/tilar.25.08dye

languages, discussing what this tells us about how we shape language and, perhaps, how language shapes us. This is followed by a look at production, and what we can learn from a language that is perceived in one modality (vision) yet seems to be produced using another modality (proprioception). As we do so, we attempt to relate what we have learned about sign language comprehension and production systems to the challenges deaf children may face in acquiring a visual language via social interaction.

Overview

Spoken languages are audio-visual languages that can be perceived by both sight and sound. The primary articulators are the lips, teeth and tongue, and the arrangements of these to produce different speech sounds results in both an acoustic signal (the speech sound itself) and a correlated visual signal (the visible arrangement of the articulators). In contrast, signed languages (excluding those used by deafblind individuals) must be perceived using vision alone – the movement of the primary articulators does not produce a corresponding auditory signal, even if one could be perceived by deaf individuals. In production, both spoken and signed languages use motor systems (moving the lips and tongue, or the hands and face). For a speaker there is access to the sound of her own voice, allowing for a clear feedback loop between the comprehension and production systems. Conversely, the visual system provides less overlap between comprehension and production for signers: visual feedback when producing signs is very different from visual input from another person's production, e.g., hand orientation and visual angle. Further, visual input during sign production is more limited compared to comprehension resulting in no clear mapping between sign comprehension and sign production (Watkins & Thompson, 2017; Emmorey, Bosworth, & Kraljic, 2009).

Children acquiring a signed language as their first language acquire it with the same ease and along the same general timeline as children acquiring a spoken language (e.g. Caselli & Volterra, 1994; Newport & Meier, 1985; Pettito & Marentette, 1991; Ross & Newport, 1996; Singleton & Newport, 2004). Nevertheless, as described above, they experience a unique set of circumstances when learning a visual language. Thus, social interaction must be altered in order to accommodate visual input (see Chapter 2 by Harris & Clibbens on interaction and Chapter 3 by van den Bogaerde & Baker on turn-taking strategies, this volume), and normal developmental milestones related to vision may need to be reached before certain aspects of using a visual language can be employed (e.g., joint attention and early visual processing). Signs are more iconic (visually motivated) than spoken words, and this might positively (or negatively) influence language development. Finally, hand-eye coordination and mapping visual comprehension onto motor output presents unique challenges in production.

It is unclear how these factors related to acquiring a visual language might influence language development. Below we describe the acquisition of the phonetic and phonological building blocks of sign and the role of feedback on that process. We focus on the psycholinguistic processes involved in using a sign language, using this research to discuss implications for sign language development.

Seeing signs during development

Not all sources of information within the visual field receive the same degree of processing. Typically, we look at the location that contains information we consider to be important. This is because light from fixated objects is projected onto the foveal region of the retina, which contains the highest density of photoreceptors – fixated objects therefore are resolved with greater acuity than objects in the periphery. In contrast, the visual periphery is good for the detection of movement and for seeing in low light conditions.

Due to these visual limitations, if signers attend to the face of their interlocutor as we know they do (see Visual Perception of Sign Language, this chapter), then they must use their peripheral visual attention to extract salient linguistic information from the moving arms, hands, and fingers. This has consequences for acquisition, especially for those deaf children whose access to a sign language is delayed. In essence, the deaf infant must "learn to look" at sign language. This requires visual attention to be drawn towards the relevant input in the environment, and then sustained (to look **at** the signal). A child must also learn to attend appropriately – with demands that are more spatial rather than temporal. Specifically, to successfully interact the deaf child must not only keep looking but must also look in the right place – the face – using covert attentional processes to extract linguistic information from the arms and hands (looking **within** the signal). If eye gaze is directed to the hands, then it's possible that fine featural distinctions expressed on the face may be missed (see Siple, 1978, for discussion).

There is evidence that the development of these attentional processes is experience-dependent and that development is at risk in deaf children with delayed exposure to sign language (Dye & Hauser, 2014; Morford & Carlson, 2011). In other words, in addition to a possible sensitive period for native-like acquisition of ASL grammar (Boudreault & Mayberry, 2006; Mayberry, 2007), there may be a corresponding sensitive period for the cognitive skills that underpin successful language processing (see Steinberg, 2005 for discussion of cognitive skills development in spoken language).

Visual perception of sign language

To date, we know very little about the visual conditions under which deaf infants and children acquire a sign language. In other words, we know little of what the linguistic signal looks like from the child's perspective. Here we discuss studies that have explored how the human visual system operates to allow information transmitted in a sign language to be perceived.

Many of these studies have used eye-tracking techniques to determine where individuals look when they are watching sign language for the purposes of comprehension. Eye tracking allows us to study where a signer is fixating when watching sign language utterances, and thus understand which source of information requires high visual acuity for successful processing. The first study to use this approach used a head-mounted eye tracker to see where deaf signers and hearing sign naïve individuals looked when watching short, filmed narratives in British Sign Language (Agrafiotis, Canagarajah, Bull, & Dye, 2003; Agrafiotis, Canagarajah, Bull, Kyle, Seers, & Dye, 2006). The aim of this study was to develop a compression algorithm for transmission of sign language video along restricted bandwidths, with spatially selective compression dependent upon where signers look. Agrafiotis et al. (2003) reported data collected from 11 participants, including deaf signers, hearing signers, and hearing non-signers, who had been asked to watch 4 short BSL narratives while their eye gaze was tracked. They reported the vertical position of fixation over time for four example participants, claiming that signers (both deaf and hearing) looked mainly at the face (particularly the mouth) with most never looking at the hands. Non-signers, however, tended to frequently fixate on the hands. This is presumably because they believed that the handshapes contained a source of information that they could use to answer comprehension questions. It is thus unclear as to whether this reflects how sign languages drive visual fixations in the absence of comprehension, as opposed to reflecting a bias stemming from a lack of knowledge regarding information transmission in sign languages.

Of course, a deaf infant being exposed to a sign language for the first time is also unaware of where salient information is located within the visual scene and must learn how to direct attention. Ongoing research is beginning to reveal the visual properties of sign languages that attract the attention of deaf infants (Stone, Petitto, & Bosworth, 2018). This research is establishing the visual analogs of *sonority* (i.e., the most salient features of the input) and suggests that a process of perceptual narrowing (e.g., Werker & Tees, 1984; Höhle, Bijeljac-Babic, Herold, Weissenborn, & Nazzi, 2009) may result in a change in infants by 12 months such that those with no sign exposure do not show a preference for attending rhythmic signed inputs over other visual inputs.

Thus, there may be a critical period for sign exposure in which the ability to home in on the perceptually most relevant aspects of the incoming sign stream develops. In support of this, there is some longitudinal evidence that non-native signers first exposed to ASL in adolescence continue to experience comprehension deficits (Morford, 2003) and that such deficits may be driven by an overreliance on handshape during sign recognition (Morford & Carlson, 2011) as was found with sign naïve observers in the Agrafiotis et al. (2003, 2006) studies. In addition, recent work has revealed that both deaf and hearing adults who acquired ASL in infancy show an enhanced ability to allocate visual attention to the inferior visual field (where the hands are located during sign production) compared to hearing adults (Stoll & Dye, 2019).

Another eye-tracking study, also with the goal of informing the design of video communication systems for the deaf, was reported by Muir and Richardson (2005). They reported that 88% of fixations were on the face (with over 80% of those fixations being to the upper half of the face). However, there was significant inter-subject variability in this regard: whereas 5 out of 10 subjects looked at the upper face over 90% of the time, 3 subjects looked at that region less than one third of the time (with one of those three spending over 50% of the time fixating the upper body, and another spending two-thirds of the viewing time looking at the lower face (presumably the mouth). Differences in visual acuity between 30-year-olds and 80-year-olds may have contributed to the large amount of inter-individual variability in the data. However, the absence of a BSL skills assessment makes it hard to interpret the inter-individual variability, and it is possible that differences may have derived from differing levels of language fluency. Nevertheless, this study highlights the importance of sustained, focused attention when perceiving sign language. Where attention is focused during sign language comprehension is a learned behavior. In the same way that a hearing person must actively listen to a speech signal, sign language comprehension is itself an active process.

There have also now been several studies on sustained visual attention in deaf children that paint a complex picture of how this ability develops. For example, while some have argued that a lack of hearing results in visual deficits such as impaired sustained attention (Smith, Quittner, Osberger, & Miyamoto, 1998; Hoffman, Tiddens, Quittner et al., 2018) and increased distractibility (Dye & Hauser, 2014), others have suggested that these apparent deficits may be driven by lower IQ (Tharpe, Ashmead, Sladen, Ryan, & Rothpletz, 2008) or by delays in the acquisition of a natural language (Dye & Hauser, 2014).

A large number of deaf infants are not exposed to sign language until much later in development, and without explicit instruction they may not automatically attend to relevant linguistic signals produced in the visual modality. Of particular concern, is the possibility that delaying exposure to a sign language early in development may result in deficits in sustained, focused attention for those children who do not go on to successfully acquire a spoken language. When a sign language is then introduced, a language-delayed deaf child may not have the cognitive resources necessary to actively engage with linguistic signals generated in the visual modality.

More recently, an eye-tracking study by Emmorey, Thompson, and Colvin (2009) looked at the eye fixation patterns of native and beginning signers when they were watching a 'live' signer, rather than a videoed sign narrative. They used two different narratives, with one involving a large number of complex classifier constructions, signed live to participants by one of five native signers. They recorded eye fixations to the "face" or "not face" (and within the face region to "just above the face", "on/near the eyes", "on/near the mouth", or "just below the face" by 9 deaf native ASL signers and 10 hearing learners of ASL (range: 9–15 months of instruction, three-to-five ASL courses). They also noted fixations away from the face, and assigned them to one of three categories based upon what kind of construction the sign narrator was producing: a lexical sign, a fingerspelled word, or a classifier. Emmorey et al. also noted whether or not the sign narrator was "auto-fixating" their own hands when the subject's eye gaze left the face area. They reported that both deaf signers and hearing learners mostly fixated the face region for both stories (over 80% of fixations) and did not significantly differ in that regard. More fine-grained differences between proficient deaf signers and learners were noted in terms of the exact facial region they were fixating, with deaf signers more likely to fixate on or near the eyes and hearing learners more likely to fixate on or near the mouth. Gaze shifts towards the hands did not appear to be driven by linguistic complexity, but rather by auto-fixations produced by the sign narrator, with this more common for classifier constructions. Emmorey et al. argued that gaze fixation does not index sign processing difficulty. Rather, maintaining fixation on the eyes by deaf signers was argued to promote language comprehension by providing a stable perceptual image from which sign information can be extracted from within the "perceptual span" of the sign receiver. They also noted that fixations on the face region promotes processing of subtle facial features that convey grammatical information in ASL and other sign languages. Hearing learners may have fixated more on the mouth, they suggested, in an attempt to speechread and leverage spoken language knowledge to better comprehend the signed language, noting that such mouthings were more likely to be produced by sign narrators when interacting with hearing learners than with other deaf signers. While this suggests that the study sacrificed some experimental control, this study was balanced by greater ecological validity. Of particular interest is that observation of a live signer seems to have increased the number of fixations to the eyes as compared to the mouth. Although cross-linguistic differences between

ASL and BSL may have driven this effect, a more parsimonious explanation at this stage would be that social interaction requires the perceiver to make eye contact with the producer, and that even small shifts of eye gaze fixation to the mouth may be detectable.

For infants learning a spoken language a general shift in attention from the eyes to the mouth of a talker has been found at about 6 months old, as infants enter the babbling phase (Lewkowicz & Hansen-Tift, 2012). This shift in attentional focus appears to be driven by infants understanding that salient information on the talker's mouth is available as synchronous support for audio input, i.e., they do it regardless of the familiarity of the language being heard (Hillairet de Boisferon, Tift, Minar, & Lewkowicz, 2015). Interestingly, gaze tends to shift back to the eyes at about 12 months (perhaps due to the requirements of social interaction). It would be interesting, therefore, to examine the gaze patterns of children learning to sign to see how these patterns change across time (to mouth or eyes) and to determine whether or not looking patterns are correlated with language exposure (to either a signed language or spoken language, or to both).

Eye tracking approaches have provided valuable information about how signers take in linguistic signals through the visual system. There is a strong tendency to fixate the face region, with studies of live signing in ASL suggesting a strong bias for fixation on the interlocutor's eyes, and video-based studies in BSL suggesting that mouth fixations are more common. In either case, information regarding handshape and movement of the arms/wrists appears to largely occur in the inferior peripheral visual field. One reason often given for the consistent fixation on the face is that sign lexicons are distributed such that a large and varied amount of information is encoded at that location. In sign languages, the face contains not only information needed to discriminate between certain pairs of lexical items (such as the ASL signs SUCCESS and ANNOUNCE), but it also conveys grammatical information such as wh- question marking (Baker-Shenk, 1983), and also affective information about emotional state (Reilly, McIntire, & Seago, 1992). This information requires high visual acuity to make the appropriate discriminations. In parallel, it has been suggested that signs where the hands are located on the face should involve a wider range of handshapes and locations that are often perceptually similar but lexically contrastive, whereas peripheral signs should have larger movements and a smaller range of handshapes which are perceptually more distinct (Siple, 1978). An analysis of a lexical database of British Sign Language signs (Fenlon, Cormier, & Brentari, 2017) revealed that signs with marked (less common and harder to perceive) handshapes were far more likely to be articulated on the head/neck than on the torso/arm. In terms of redundancy, signs that used two hands that shared the same handshape were more common on the torso/arm than on the head/neck, with one-handed signs more often located in the latter region.

The visual periphery may have poor acuity, but it is adept at detecting and processing movement, and can also localize visual stimuli with impressive accuracy. But handshape identity is not perfectly decoded in the periphery, at least when signs are presented in isolation (Swisher, Christie, & Miller, 1989). How then do signers overcome the limitations of the human visual perceptual system in order to effortlessly comprehend linguistic information encoded within sign languages? One possibility is that the linguistic system itself undergoes structural changes as it is passed from one generation to another – over time, signs may shift to be closer to the center of fixation (increasing visual acuity at the sign location) or the number of handshapes employed may be reduced. Another possibility is that new linguistic constraints emerge – such as the symmetry and dominance constraints (Battison, 1978) – which minimize the demands on the perceptual system. The hypothesis that sign languages have evolved in order to conform to visual perceptual constraints has some limited support in the literature. Analysis of ASL data (Frishberg, 1975; Woodward, 1976) suggests that over time signs originally articulated near the abdomen have moved upwards to become more centralized. That is, they gravitate towards a sign location near the upper chest of the signer. A similar study of diachronic change in BSL (Woll, 1987) found a tendency for signs located on the head to move towards the same upper chest region. These analyses, however, have been based upon comparisons of current sign forms with pictures or written reports of what signs looked like in the past. They therefore provide only limited support for the contention that sign languages have evolved to conform to the constraints imposed by the human visual system (Siple, 1978). The advent of lexical databases – such as the BSL Sign Bank (Fenlon, Cormier, Rentelis, Schembri, Rowley, Adam, & Woll, 2014) and ASL-LEX (Caselli, Sehyr, Cohen-Goldberg, & Emmorey, 2017) will allow psycholinguists to further test these claims around sign perception and visual structure, many of which are based upon limited and selected exemplars (e.g. Siple, 1978) or accounts of language change from incomplete historical documentation (Frishberg, 1975; Woll, 1987).

In parallel with perceptually-motivated change in sign forms, an additional possibility is that the human visual system itself adapts to the demands imposed by the linguistic system to which the language learner is exposed in order to help an individual signer accommodate and identify detailed information in the visual periphery. There is some evidence that visual attention may be allocated away from the location of eye gaze fixation in signers, in a way that is not observed in users of spoken languages. Specifically, it has been suggested that native users of ASL have an inferior visual field advantage that could potentially ease processing of information in the lower periphery by decreasing the size of perceptive visual fields and thereby increasing effective acuity (Dye, 2016). This conclusion was formulated based upon a reanalysis of the errors in a Useful Field of View (UFOV) task (Dye, Hauser, & Bavelier, 2009). The UFOV requires observers to apprehend a complex visual scene (without any eye movement) and indicate the location of a peripheral target. This paradigm has been used to demonstrate a superior visual field bias in typically hearing individuals – targets in the superior visual field are more easily detected (Feng & Spence, 2014). The reanalysis of the errors revealed that, on incorrect trials, typically hearing non-signers were more likely to guess that the target appeared at an inferior visual field location than an upper visual field location – that is, they were biased to guess that the target appeared at a location where hearing observers typically perform more poorly, also reflecting a superior visual field bias. In signers of ASL, however, the distribution of errors was significantly less biased towards the inferior visual field, regardless of hearing status. This, paradoxically, suggests a shift in the focus of attention towards lower parts of the visual field attributable to use of a sign language.

Another study computed thresholds for direction-of-motion discrimination in deaf signers, hearing signers, and hearing non-signers (Bosworth & Dobkins, 2002). They reported that the deaf signers had lower thresholds for targets in the inferior visual field than for those in the superior visual field. That is, compared to their hearing peers, deaf native users of a sign language could detect direction-of-motion in the inferior visual field when a lower percentage of dots were moving coherently. For both groups of hearing participants there was no bias toward either the inferior or superior visual field on their task. While they concluded that the effect was driven by deafness and not by using a sign language, their sample of hearing signers reported using ASL on only a weekly or daily basis. It is possible that frequent use of sign language, rather than age of acquisition or fluency, is the driving force behind a redistribution of visual attention to the inferior visual field. More recent work has indeed suggested that both hearing and deaf signers who acquired ASL in infancy have a bias towards attending to the inferior visual field (Stoll & Dye, 2019), implying a causative role for sign language exposure. That is, the ability to maintain joint eye gaze with an interlocutor while at the same time processing signs produced in the inferior visual field is experience-dependent. What we do not yet know is whether there is a sensitive period within which exposure to a sign language must occur for this pattern to occur. Again, this has important implications for sign language acquisition in deaf children. Delayed exposure to sign may result in a visual attentional system that cannot support extraction of handshape information from the periphery, requires the perceiver to decide between missing phonological or morphological information provided by handshape, or shifting their gaze away from the face more often. The eye tracking data from Emmorey et al. (2009) suggest that most adult sign novices do the former. This, in turn, may limit the amount of information uptake from the sign language input, and/or increase the cognitive demands and effort of comprehending the language in those with delayed exposure to sign. However, we know almost nothing about eye movements or visual attention changes in fluent signers who acquired a sign language late in development. The implications of delayed ASL acquisition, in this regard, are therefore unknown.

The above section has summarized what we know about how the visual system processes visual language, how this develops in native signers, and how in non-native signers these processes may be sensitive to early disruptions related to wider cognitive and attentional differences. During sign language development, once children have established that signs have meanings they can then use their cognitive systems to break into vocabulary by focusing attention on different cues in the sign. One such cue that has been proposed to help sign language learning is *iconicity*, or the meaningful links between form and meaning, in a visual language.

Visually motivated sign language lexicons can influence language processing in adults. Specifically, iconicity, has been shown to play a role in language processing both for comprehension (Thompson, Vinson, & Vigliocco, 2009) and production (Vinson, Thompson, Skinner, & Vigliocco, 2015). While a serious exploration of iconic (sound-symbolic) mappings in spoken language has only recently begun, the literature for spoken language acquisition clearly favors a role for iconicity in spoken language acquisition (Dingemanse, Blasi, Lupyan, Christiansen, & Monaghan, 2015; Perniss, Thompson, & Vigliocco, 2010; Perry, Perlman, Winter, Massaro, & Lupyan, 2018), while research on the role of iconicity in sign language acquisition has been more mixed (for discussion see Thompson, 2011; Ortega, 2017).

One longitudinal study of four deaf children examined ASL sign errors that were observed from as early as 8 months and continuing as late as 17 months (Meier, Mauk, Cheek, & Moreland, 2008) and found that single sign errors in a child's production do not tend to be more iconic than the adult forms. Instead errors exhibit normal patterns of phonological reduction and substitution of less marked features. Meier et al. conclude that factors such as phonological complexity are more important than iconicity in acquisition.

In a study of adult sign learning, Ortega and Morgan (2015) found that iconicity interfered with accurate articulation of signs in a sign repetition task for beginning adult L2 learners of BSL. They suggested that L2 learners remembered the iconic aspects of iconic signs, leading to non-specific learning of a sign's phonological features and therefore subsequent misarticulation during production. Interestingly, Ortega and Morgan showed that errors in sign production for L2 learners are iconic approximations of the sign, running counter to the conclusions of Meier et al. (2008). However, similar to Meier et al., they reported that phonology was the largest predictor of accuracy. Specifically, some phonological aspects of a sign are easier to reproduce than others, with handshape the most difficult, followed by path movement, then palm orientation, and finally sign location.

Clearly, other aspects of sign language such as the phonological makeup of an individual sign can influence acquisition (particularly in production). However, children may nevertheless also make use of iconic form-meaning mappings to enter the language system. In support of this, research that seeks to take into account several different factors alongside of iconicity has shown that iconicity is important for acquisition over and above these other factors.

Based on parental reports of the MacArthur Bates British Sign Language Communicative Development Inventory (BSL CDI), signing children were found to be significantly better at both comprehending and producing more iconic signs, compared to less iconic signs, even after accounting for effects of phonological complexity and familiarity (i.e., subjective frequency based on ratings; Thompson, Vinson, Woll, & Vigliocco, 2012). In a replication study in American Sign Language (ASL) using the ASL CDI (Caselli & Pyers, 2017), iconicity was again found to be a factor in earlier acquisition of signs with the additional finding that alongside iconicity, neighborhood density and subjective lexical frequency also predicted sign acquisition. Thus, the evidence suggests that iconicity may be only one of many interacting factors that drive acquisition.

Individual sign variables such as phonological complexity and neighborhood density are not the only relevant aspects of acquisition that may influence how effective a child is at taking advantage of iconic aspects of signs. In spoken language acquisition, a much debated finding is a 'noun-bias' which claims that children tend to learn nouns more quickly compared to other words such as verbs, likely because they refer to more easily understood and accessed concepts for more concrete objects (Gentner, 2006). While the noun bias has been found in many languages, there is sufficient conflicting evidence (e.g., in Korean, Mandarin and Turkish) to suggest that the noun bias may be language dependent (see Waxman, Fu, Arunachalam, Leddon, Geraghty, & Song, 2013, for discussion).

For sign language learning, iconicity may play a role in driving a preference for action words (verbs) over more concrete object words in acquisition. Using a picture description task, Ortega, Sumer and Ozyurek (2017) recently found that Turkish preschool and school-age deaf signing children favored sign variants representing actions associated with their referent (e.g., a writing hand for the sign PEN), while adults preferred variants representing the perceptual features of those objects (e.g. an upward index finger representing a thin, elongated object for the sign PEN). Ortega et al. suggest that when children are confronted with two variants for the same concept, they initially prefer action-based variants because these variants provide the opportunity to link a linguistic label to familiar schemas based on their action/motor experiences. These results, however, may not be indicative of the order of learning since it is not clear whether children comprehended both variants for a given sign.

Finally, Lu, and Thompson (2017) recently showed that, for adult L2 learners, the learning environment makes a difference in the effectiveness of iconicity in sign learning. In a word-learning experiment, the degree of similarity between phonological properties of signs and semantic categories of referents was manipulated (e.g., signs produced on the sides of the head were taught within similar categories of animals with antlers such as deer, moose, cow). Overall, iconic signs were more helpful than arbitrary ones for learning regardless of learning environment. However, learners were less accurate and slower at learning signs that had greater phonological similarity (i.e., both signs sharing place of articulation), but not when signs were semantically similar (i.e., both signs referring to similar objects). These results indicate that iconicity can hinder learning in some contexts.

There is still more to be done in order to fully understand the role of iconicity in sign language learning and acquisition. One question that has recently begun to be addressed is the role of caregiver input on the benefits of iconicity in sign acquisition. Perniss, Lu, Morgan, and Vigliocco (2018) asked BSL signers to imagine playing with their child using specific toys that were either present or not. They found that iconic signs were more likely to be modified in infant-directed language in a way that highlights the meaningful link between the sign and its meaning. The findings suggest that caregivers are aware of iconicity and take advantage of it to bootstrap a child into the language.

With this section on comprehension of signs completed we now turn to the other side of the coin in terms of language development, that of language production.

Production of a visual language

Turning to articulation, several studies have examined what the production of sign languages tells us about the processing architecture for visual languages like ASL and BSL. Unlike spoken languages, the signer's experience of the language they produce is qualitatively different from that of their interlocutor. While a speaker has a proprioceptive experience due to movement of the speech articulators, the acoustic product of that articulation is also experienced via the speaker's own auditory system in a qualitatively similar way to how it is experienced by an interlocutor. For a signed language, however, the visual experience of signing is very different depending upon whether a signer is the producer or the comprehender of an utterance. Therefore, while sign production is perceived through the visual modality, it has been suggested that the signer's experience is much more proprioceptive than it is for a speaker of a spoken language. A study by Emmorey, Bosworth, and Kralic (2009) sought to determine how much visual feedback was available to signers when they looked at ASL numeral signs. Thirteen fluent ASL signers (12 deaf and 1 hearing) were asked to identify ASL numerals ('6' through '9') presented from either a first-person perspective (as if produced by themselves) or a third-person perspective (as if produced by another signer). These stimuli were presented at one of two locations – either 14.4 or 45.0 degrees of visual angle from the participant's point of fixation. Analysis of identification accuracy revealed that the first-person perspective was harder than a third-person perspective, and that peripheral stimuli were harder to identify than more centrally located stimuli. Interestingly, they reported that accuracy at identifying numeral signs from a first-person perspective was relatively unaffected by eccentricity (how far the sign was from eye fixation), suggesting that this reflected experience with perceiving one's own sign production in the far periphery. It is important to note, however, that while better than chance (25%), identification accuracy for first-person perspective stimuli (45–90%) was worse than for third-person stimuli (82–97%) emphasizing the fact that visual feedback in sign languages may be less reliable than auditory feedback for spoken languages.[1] In the same article, Emmorey and colleagues asked 28 deaf ASL signers to imitate signs from Russian Sign Language. These signs were selected to be hard to produce and required the production of handshapes not attested in ASL, unusual handshape combinations, and location-movement articulations that were not allowed in ASL. The ASL signers produced these signs while wearing safety glasses that altered how much visual feedback could be obtained during imitation (normal, blurred, or no feedback). The amount/quality of visual feedback had little-to-no effect on the accuracy of sign imitation, suggesting that visual feedback does not operate in the same way in sign languages as auditory feedback does for spoken languages.

Further, with respect to visual monitoring, Emmorey, Korpics, and Petronio (2009) reported a study of sign production in individuals with Usher Syndrome – a condition that, in addition to deafness, is characterized by a progressive reduction in the size of the perceivable visual field. They recruited 15 deaf ASL signers to participate in their study: five typically sighted individuals, five who had Usher Syndrome and experienced "tunnel vision", and five with Usher Syndrome and no functional vision. These signers were asked to interact with another signer in a discussion of life experiences regarding interpreters, and to produce a monologue following the script of a short story. Around four minutes of signing was selected from each participant and they calculated the percentage of time that signs were produced within a "box" bounded vertically by the top of the signer's head and the top one-third of the signer's chest. Signers with tunnel vision produced more signs

---

1. Note, however, that the ASL numerals SIX through NINE are very similar phonologically. It is unclear what a speaker's performance would look like if listening to similar sounding words in a noisy environment.

in the face area than did the other two groups, who did not differ in this regard. In addition, dialogues resulted in more signs located nearer the face than monologues, regardless of signer group. Planned comparisons revealed that signers with tunnel vision signed nearer the face more for dialogues than for monologues. The researchers argued that increased signing near the face by tunnel vision signers (for both monologues and dialogues) supported the hypothesis that they use visual feedback for monitoring sign production.

It is well known that speech production can be distorted via manipulation of auditory feedback. A study by Emmorey, Gertsberg, Korpics, and Wright (2009) sought to determine whether sign production is disturbed when visual feedback is manipulated. They reported data from five native or near-native signers who produced short ASL sentences in five different conditions: "normal" signing, informal signing, "shouting", signing with a restricted field of view, and blindfolded signing. As they produced the sentences, an Optotrak motion capture system was used to record movement of the dominant hand (with IR emitting diodes attached to the signer's hand, shoulder and temple). Blindfolded signing resulted in signs with longer durations, but had no effect on location, size of signing space, or sign velocity. When signing with a restricted field of view, signs were restricted in the vertical dimension, although the median height of signing was not displaced. They argued that visual feedback was being used to calibrate the size of signing space within which signs were articulated, although it did not serve to keep hands moving within the visual field of the signer. Conversely, they argued, it seemed unlikely that visual feedback was providing an error signal with which monitoring could be facilitated within the language production system.

Together, these studies suggest that visual feedback is available to signers, although it is unclear to what extent it is used as a way to monitor production for possible errors. However, across all of these studies, whereas Emmorey and colleagues manipulated the amount of visual feedback available to their participants, or studied individuals with atypical vision, they did not alter the timing of that feedback. For speech, delayed auditory feedback is known to impair production and can result in stutter-like symptoms.

Importantly, during language development children acquiring spoken languages get full access to auditory feedback of their own voices. However because many sign locations are not in the signer's visual field (e.g., a sign on the signer's own head) in some cases the child has to produce a sign with little or no visual feedback. Indeed, deaf mothers appear to implicitly acknowledge the saliency of proprioceptive feedback for sign production, and have been observed to mold the handshapes of their infants as corrective input (Pizer, Meier, & Shaw Points, 2011).

Data suggests that, at least during development, visual feedback of one's own signs is useful. First, although we know of no studies to date, there is anecdotal evidence that young children auto-fixate their hands during sign production to a much greater degree than adults do. This suggests a greater reliance on visual feedback during language development, allied to child-directed corrective feedback. In support of this, Boyes-Braem (1990) argued that patterns of handshape development could be predicted by available visual and proprioceptive feedback during production alongside the motoric and phonological complexity of the sign. Further, there is evidence that young signers make more self-articulation errors with handshapes that are made at locations in peripheral compared with central vision (Ortega & Morgan, 2010).

Another feature of signing that differs from speech is the size of the major articulators. Young children's gross movement development influences their articulation of signs. Two characteristics noted in the literature (Meier, 2006) are proximalization (where distal joint articulation in signs changes to joints closer to the body) and sympathy (one-handed signs get changed into two-handed ones). There do not appear to be comparable phenomena in spoken development.

Related to this are differences in signer handedness that could influence how individual signs are learned. During production, signers make use of both hands as articulators. Signs are produced with one hand, two symmetrical hands (that share handshape and movement), or two asymmetrical hands (with different handshapes). Signers can be either right or left-hand dominant, meaning that their primary articulator (the only one used for one-handed signs) can be either the right or left hand. Importantly, hand dominance while signing has no consequences for sign meaning. Watkins and Thompson (2017) found differences in processing for adults related to their handedness and the corresponding handedness of a sign model. Using a picture-sign matching task, both left- and right-hand dominant signers were found to be faster to respond ("yes" the sign and picture match) when viewing right-handed signers (suggesting a frequency effect). However, this was not the case when they viewed signs with two asymmetrical hands. For these phonologically more complex signs, signers were faster to respond when they shared hand dominance with the sign model. Crucially, during language development, a child must learn to map input from signers onto their own body schema (right or left-handed). There are no studies investigating how handedness might impact acquisition. Future research could investigate the relative age of acquisition of signs, particularly of more phonologically complex signs, in development for right-and left-handed children.

Handedness differences in signing demonstrate only one aspect of the complicated task that children face during sign language acquisition. More generally, children must solve a complicated mapping problem by mapping the signs they see onto the signs they will produce. Recently, Shield and Meier (2018) investigated possible imitation strategies that signers might adopt during development to solve this mapping problem. Making use of existing data, they found that children initially use a visual matching strategy in which they reproduce what they see from their own perspective. A visual matching strategy can be seen in children's movement and palm orientation errors, e.g., a sign beginning on the signer's body and moving away from the body would be reproduced by a child with a location away from the body and a movement in towards the body. Shield and Meier further report that typically developing children switch to a mirroring strategy sometime in the second year of life. By contrast, children and adults with autism spectrum disorder (ASD) appear to use the visual matching strategy well into childhood or even adulthood. Overall, this research adds to our understanding of naturally occurring movement errors reported for young, typical deaf children acquiring sign (Siedlecki & Bonvillian, 1993; Marentette & Mayberry, 2000; Meier, 2006; Morgan, Barrett-Jones, & Stoneham, 2007) which cannot distinguish between errors due to motor control, and those errors that arise due to mapping errors.

Another source of information about the sign production system lives in "slips of the hand". Analogous to slips of the tongue in speech, these production errors have been used to elucidate mechanisms of sign language production. The seminal work on slips of the hand was published by Newkirk, Klima, Pedersen, and Bellugi (1980), who analyzed a corpus of 131 slips of the hand in ASL (77 were from videotapes of narrative signing, and 54 were reported observations from informants). A notation system was used to annotate each of the 131 slips. Based upon this annotation, slips were categorized according to (a) which parameters were involved, (b) whether the slip was a metathesis, anticipation, or perseveration. and (c) the degree of separation between the two signs involved in the slip. In addition, native signers considered whether the resultant slips were real ASL signs, possible but unattested signs, or impossible in ASL. Whole sign slips (9 out of 131) were less common than slips involving an exchange of values for a single feature. Within these, exchanges of handshape were the most common (65), followed by location (13) and movement (11). The occurrences of slips that were not allowed in ASL were infrequent (5 out of 131). Newkirk and colleagues argued that feature exchanges provided evidence for signs being componential and not holistic, and that infrequent illegal forms suggested that rule-bound sublexical parameters are actually involved in sign production, and not merely a byproduct of way in which signs and sign errors were analyzed.

While it is important to note that over 40% of the production errors analyzed in Newkirk et al. were not actually observed by the researchers, and were based upon anecdotal reports from individuals associated with their lab, it must also be considered that this was seminal work in the field. In addition, the findings have been validated in a subsequent study of production errors in German Sign Language (DGS) by Hohenberger, Happ, and Leuniger (2002). This group used language elicitation approaches to increase the likelihood of slips of the hand in a sample of ten adult deaf signers. They were shown fourteen picture stories and asked to retell the stories in DGS. A range of approaches were employed to increase cognitive load and induce errors, such as signing stories based upon muddled picture sequences, signing under pressure, and cumulative picture repetition. Slips of the hand were identified by a deaf linguist fluent in DGS, and categorized on the basis of the slip type (anticipation, substitution, blend, deletion, etc.), the linguistic entity involved in the slip (feature, morpheme, word, phrase), whether the signer corrected themselves (yes, no) and when the correction occurred (before word, within word, after word, delayed). The most common slip types observed (over 203 tokens) were perseverations (22.1%), anticipations (21.7%), semantic substitutions (18.7%), and blends (15.7%). Words were the most common loci of slips, followed by phonological features. In terms of the timing of repairs when slips occur, 59.1% of such repairs in the corpus occurred before or within a word. This contrasts with the repair timing reported for a corpus of spoken Dutch slips of the tongue: only 23% were corrected within a word (and 0% before). No inferential statistics are provided by Hohenberger et al., but a chi-square analysis based upon reported frequency data suggests that an equivalent allocation of errors to different timing categories across the two languages can be rejected as a plausible hypothesis. On the basis of this latter repair timing data, the researchers argued that the timing of repair behavior in DGS (compared to spoken Dutch) is best explained as resulting from the longer syllables in DGS words (which they argue are mostly monosyllabic) taking longer to articulate. With an internal error monitor in the language processing system (Levelt, 1989) that has the same temporal properties, errors are likely to be detected earlier within a DGS sign than they would be for a word in spoken Dutch. However, interpretation of repair timing differences is complicated because hearing speakers of Dutch were compared with deaf signers of DGS. A better design would include CODAs to control for potential deaf–hearing differences not related to language modality, and to permit collection of spoken and signed repair data within the same individuals. It is also unclear whether the "earlier" detection of DGS slips (and their subsequent repair) is due to longer articulation times in DGS compared to spoken Dutch, or because the production signal is faster to arrive at the monitor (assuming that it is kinesthetic or proprioceptive) compared to the speed at which auditory feedback is received. Nevertheless, this provides intriguing evidence to suggest that aspects of the language production system may be unmalleable, resulting in processing differences when language structures differ.

Another study to use production errors as a window into the language processing architecture was reported by Vinson, Thompson, Skinner, Fox, and Vigliocco (2010), who sought to determine whether mouthings (as opposed to mouth gestures) and manual components of BSL share the same semantic representation, or whether their production stems from activation of two separate representational systems. They made use of picture naming and word naming tasks to bring about errors, and examined the co-occurrence of mouthing and manual component errors, reasoning that if the production of mouthings and manual sign components is the result of two separate production systems, then co-occurrence of semantic errors in the two channels should be relatively uncommon. Fifteen native BSL signers (eight deaf and seven hearing) were presented with lists of semantically related or unrelated pictures or words, and asked to name the pictures or translate the words in BSL. Vinson and colleagues analyzed the distribution of errors across different categories for both mouthings and manual sign components. In their error corpus, there were 190 manual semantic errors, and 70 semantic errors in mouthing. Importantly, they reported that only 19 errors contained both a manual and a mouthing semantic error – that is, semantic errors tended to occur in either one modality (mouthing, manual) or the other. Vinson et al. argued that if the two modalities shared the same lexico-semantic representation, then the co-occurrence of mouthing and manual semantic errors should be much higher, and that therefore it is likely that the mouthing component is represented separately.

A related phenomenon is "tip of the fingers" (TOF) states, that provide information about retrieval processes during language production. A study by Thompson, Emmorey, and Gollan (2005) sought to examine the existence and structure of TOF states in a sample of 33 deaf ASL signers. An elicitation task was used, with signers asked to name twenty pictures of famous faces – to induce fingerspell TOFs – and to translate written English words into ASL – to induce lexical TOFs. Participants produced a total of 79 TOFs –24 were lexical, and 55 were fingerspells. Of the lexical TOFs most (22/24) were for proper names, and, for 19 of the 24, participants could recall some phonological parameters (handshape, location, orientation, or movement). Indeed, for 10 out of these 19, participants recalled 3 out of the 4 parameters, failing to retrieve only one. Handshape, location and orientation were equally likely to be recalled, but movement was significantly less likely to be recalled than other parameters. An analysis of chance performance suggested that reports were the result of incomplete lexical access to a target sign, and not guessing. Thompson and colleagues argued that this provided evidence for a dissociation between semantics and phonology, because the iconic components of signs were not more likely to be retrieved during incomplete access (although only one example, SWITZERLAND, is provided in the article). TOFs were similar to tips of the tongue in that proper nouns were the most common lexical targets when incomplete access occurred. The data also suggest that sign production appears to be a heavily parallel process, with handshape, location and orientation being recalled at first, and movement then being accessed last, resulting in many examples where three parameters were recalled, but one was elusive.

While we know that children acquiring a sign language make production errors (Bellugi & Klima, 1991; Boyes-Braem, 1990; Crowson, 1994; Hoffmeister & Wilbur, 1980; McIntire, 1977; Newport & Meier, 1985; Schick, 1990), past studies have been conducted in the context of acquisition rather than language processing per se. We therefore know next to nothing about the type and pattern of slips of the hand and tip-of-the-finger states in children acquiring a sign language and what that reveals about how they are coping with the processing demands of the language.

Summary

To summarize, what we have learned about sign language comprehension and production has several potential implications for sign language acquisition by deaf and hearing infants and children. Firstly, infants must learn to look in the right place. While ongoing research is still establishing the critical period during which infants learn to distinguish between linguistic and non-linguistic visual inputs, we know that adult signers exposed to a sign language from birth are able to look at an interlocutor's face while processing sign input from the inferior (lower) visual field. This latter redistribution of visual attention seems to be present for both hearing and deaf adults, suggesting that it is driven by exposure to sign language and not by deafness. Just how much exposure is required, and at what age, is the subject of ongoing research. Eye tracking data suggests that adults who are beginning signers are able to maintain fixation on the face (unlike sign naïve observers), but the extent to which they can extract necessary linguistic parameters from the inferior visual field is unknown.

We know that iconicity appears to be more prevalent in signed than in spoken languages, and, again, this seems to have implications for acquisition. While at one time iconicity was believed to be epiphenomenal, more recent work has revealed that the early vocabulary of young deaf children has an over-representation of iconic signs and, importantly, that native signing caregivers are sensitive to this and use iconicity to help bootstrap their children into language. Iconicity also affects the other side of the language processing coin – production. A child's early sign productions may be heavily influenced by iconicity, at the expense of accurate phonological production (for the contra argument see the analysis in Meier, Mauk, Cheek, & Moreland, 2008). Indeed, errors in sign production are typical of fluent adult language production also. There are some interesting differences between production errors in speech and sign, and repair processes following errors may have surface differences that still reflect the same underlying processing architecture. While tolerance for production errors in young children acquiring a sign language is important, there is a paucity of data on what typical child sign errors look like, and how deaf caregivers help a child to repair those errors, if at all.

In this chapter, we have attempted to derive implications for sign language acquisition from psycholinguistic studies of sign comprehension and production. We caution, however, that inferring acquisition processes from adult processing data is fraught with dangers of overextension and overgeneralization. We note that there is a growing trend, at least in the United States, to promote early exposure to sign language for deaf children born to hearing parents. These parents are in desperate need of information about the linguistic environments that their child needs, as well as about what is typical or atypical in terms of sign comprehension and production. A focus in the past on language processing in adults exposed to a sign language from birth has revealed a great deal about the nature of language generally, and the specific processing demands of sign languages in particular. However, more work is needed to address the developmental psycholinguistics of sign language comprehension and production if we are to be able to provide sound information to parents and educators.

References

Agrafiotis, D., Canagarajah, N., Bull, D. R., & Dye, M. (2003). Perceptually optimised sign language video coding based on eye tracking analysis. *Electronics Letters* 39(24), 1703–1705. https://doi.org/10.1049/el:20031140

Agrafiotis, D., Canagarajah, N., Bull, D. R., Kyle, J., Seers, H., & Dye, M. (2006). A perceptually optimised video coding system for sign language communication at low bit rates. *Signal Processing: Image Communication* 21(7), 531–549.

Baker-Shenk, C. (1983). *A micro-analysis of the non-manual components of questions in American Sign Language*. Berkeley, CA: University of California.

Battison, R. (1978). *Lexical borrowing in American Sign Language*. Silver Spring, MD: Linstok Press.

Bellugi, U., & Klima, E. (1991). What the hands reveal about the brain. In D. S. Martin (Ed.), *Advances in cognition, education and deafness*. Washington, DC: Gallaudet University Press.

Bosworth, R. G., & Dobkins, K. R. (2002). Visual field asymmetries for motion processing in deaf and hearing signers. *Brain & Cognition* 49, 170–181. https://doi.org/10.1006/brcg.2001.1498

Boudreault, P., & Mayberry, R. L. (2006). Grammatical processing in American Sign Language: Age of first-language acquisition effects in relation to syntactic structure. *Language & Cognitive Processes* 21(5), 608–635. https://doi.org/10.1080/01690960500139363

Boyes-Braem, P. (1990). The acquisition of handshapes in American Sign Language. In V. Volterra, & C. Erting (Eds), *From gesture to language in deaf and hearing children*. New York, NY: Springer. https://doi.org/10.1007/978-3-642-74859-2_10

Caselli M. C., & Volterra, V. (1994). From communication to language in hearing and deaf children. In V. Volterra, & C. Erting (Eds), *From gesture to language in hearing and deaf children* (pp. 263–278). New York, NY: Springer.

Caselli, N. K., & Pyers, J. E. (2017). The road to language learning is not entirely iconic: Iconicity, neighborhood density, and frequency facilitate sign language acquisition. *Psychological Science* 28(7), 979–987. https://doi.org/10.1177/0956797617700498

Caselli, N. K., Sehyr, Z. S., Cohen-Goldberg A. M., & Emmorey, K. (2017). ASL-LEX: A lexical database of American Sign Language. *Behaviour Research Methods* 49(2):784–801. https://doi.org/10.3758/s13428-016-0742-0.

Conlin, K. E., Mirus, G. R., Mauk, C., & Meier, R. P. (2000). The acquisition of first signs: Place, handshape, and movement. In C. Chamberlain, J. P. Morford, & R. I. Mayberry (Eds.), *Language acquisition by eye* (pp. 51–70). Mahwah, NJ: Lawrence Erlbaum Associates.

Crowson, K. (1994). Errors made by deaf children acquiring sign language. *Early Child Development & Care* 99, 63–78. https://doi.org/10.1080/0300443940990106

Dingemanse, M., Blasi, D. E., Lupyan, G., Christiansen, M. H., & Monaghan, P. (2015). Arbitrariness, iconicity, and systematicity in language. *Trends in Cognitive Sciences* 19(10), 603–615. https://doi.org/10.1016/j.tics.2015.07.013

Dye, M. W. G., Hauser, P. C., & Bavelier, D. (2009). Is visual attention in deaf individuals enhanced or deficient? The case of the Useful Field of View. *PLoS One* 4(5), e5640. https://doi.org/10.1371/journal.pone.0005640

Dye, M. W. G., & Hauser, P. C. (2014). Sustained attention, selective attention and cognitive control in deaf and hearing children. *Hearing Research* 309, 94–102. https://doi.org/10.1016/j.heares.2013.12.001

Dye, M. W. G. (2016). Response bias reveals enhanced attention to inferior visual field in signers of American Sign Language. *Experimental Brain Research* 234(4), 1067–1076. https://doi.org/10.1007/s00221-015-4530-3

Emmorey, K. (2002). *Language, cognition, and the brain: Insights from sign language research.* Mahwah, NJ: Lawrence Erlbaum Associates.

Emmorey, K. (2000). *The signs of language revisited: An anthology to honor Ursula Bellugi and Edward Klima.* Mahwah, NJ: Lawrence Erlbaum Associates.

Emmorey, K., Bosworth, R., & Kraljic, T. (2009). Visual feedback and self-monitoring of sign language. *Journal of Memory & Language* 61(3), 398–411. https://doi.org/10.1016/j.jml.2009.06.001

Emmorey K., Gertsberg, N., Korpics, F., & Wright, C. E. (2009). The influence of visual feedback and register changes on sign language production: A kinematic study with deaf signers. *Applied Psycholinguistics* 30, 187–203. https://doi.org/10.1017/S0142716408090085

Emmorey, K., Korpics, F., & Petronio, K. (2009). The use of visual feedback during signing: Evidence from signers with impaired vision. *The Journal of Deaf Studies & Deaf Education* 14(1), 99–104. https://doi.org/10.1093/deafed/enn020

Emmorey, K., Thompson, R. L., & Colvin, R. (2009). Eye gaze during comprehension of American Sign Language by native and beginning signers. *Journal of Deaf Studies and Deaf Education* 14(2), 237–243. https://doi.org/10.1093/deafed/enn037

Feng, J., & Spence, I. (2014). Upper visual field advantage in localizing a target among distractors. *i-Perception* 5, 97–100. https://doi.org/10.1068/i0625rep

Fenlon, J., Cormier, K., & Brentari, D. (2017). The phonology of sign languages. In S. J. Hannahs, & A. Bosch (Eds.), *The Routledge handbook of phonological theory.* London: Routledge.

Fenlon, J., Cormier, K., Rentelis, R., Schembri, A., Rowley, K., Adam, R., & Woll, B. (2014). *BSL SignBank: A lexical database of British Sign Language* (first ed.). London: Deafness, Cognition and Language Research Centre, University College London.

Frishberg, N. (1975). Arbitrariness and iconicity: Historical change in American Sign Language. *Language* 51(3), 696–719.   https://doi.org/10.2307/412894

Gentner, D. (2006). Why verbs are hard to learn. In K. A. Hirsh-Pasek & R. M. Golinkoff (Eds.), *Action meets word: How children learn verbs* (pp. 544–564). New York, NY: Oxford University Press.   https://doi.org/10.1093/acprof:oso/9780195170009.003.0022

Hillairet de Boisferon, A., Tift, A. H., Minar, N. J, & Lewkowicz, D. J. (2015). Selective attention to a talker's mouth in infancy: role of audiovisual temporal synchrony and linguistic experience. *Developmental Science* 20(3), e12381.   https://doi.org/10.1111/desc.12381

Hoffman, M., Tiddens, E., Quittner, A. L. and the CDaCI Investigative Team. (2018). Comparisons of visual attention in school-age children with cochlear implants versus hearing peers and normative data. *Hearing Research* 359, 91–100.
https://doi.org/10.1016/j.heares.2018.01.002

Hoffmeister, R., & Wilbur, R. (1980). The acquisition of sign language. In H. Lane & F. Grosjean (Eds.), *Recent perspectives on American Sign Language*. Hillsdale, NJ: Lawrence Erlbaum Associates.

Hohenberger, A., Happ, D., & Leuniger, H. (2002). Modality-dependent aspects of sign language production: Evidence from slips of the hands and their repairs in German Sign Language. In R. P. Meier, K. A. Cormier, & D. Quinto-Pozos (Eds.), *Modality and structure in signed and spoken language* (pp. 112–142). Cambridge: Cambridge University Press.
https://doi.org/10.1017/CBO9780511486777.006

Höhle, B., Bijeljac-Babic, R., Herold, B., Weissenborn, J., & Nazzi, T. (2009). Language specific prosodic preferences during the first year of life. Evidence from German and French infants. *Infant Behavioural Development* 32, 262–274.
https://doi.org/10.1016/j.infbeh.2009.03.004

Kyle, J. G., & Woll, B. (1985). *Sign language: The study of deaf people and their language*. New York, NY: Cambridge University Press.

Levelt, P. (1989). *Speaking: From intention to articulation*. Cambridge, MA: The MIT Press.

Lewkowicz, D. J., & Hansen-Tift, A. M. (2012). Infants deploy selective attention to the mouth of a talking face when learning speech. *Proceedings of the National Academy of Sciences* 109(5), 1431–1436.   https://doi.org/10.1073/pnas.1114783109

Lu, J., & Thompson, R. L. (2017). Different word learning contexts modulate the learnability of iconic signs. Paper presented at the *8th Conference of the International Society for Gesture Studies – Gesture and Diversity*. Cape Town.

Marentette, P. F., & Mayberry, R. I. (2000). Principles for an emerging phonological system: A case study of early ASL acquisition. In C. Chamberlain, J. P. Morford, & R. I. Mayberry (Eds), *Language Acquisition by Eye* (pp. 71–90). Mahwah, NJ: Lawrence Erlbaum Associates.

Marschark, M., Siple, P., Lillo-Martin, D., Campbell, R., & Everhart, V. S. (1997). *Relations of language and thought: The view from sign language and deaf children*. New York, NY: Oxford University Press.

Marschark, M., & Hauser, P. C. (Eds.). (2008). *Deaf cognition: foundations and outcomes*. New York, NY: Oxford University Press.
https://doi.org/10.1093/acprof:oso/9780195368673.001.0001

Mayberry, R. (2007). When timing is everything: Age of first-language acquisition effects on second-language learning. *Applied Psycholinguistics* 28(3), 537–549. https://doi.org/10.1017/S0142716407070294

McIntire, M. L. (1977). The acquisition of American Sign Language hand configurations. *Sign Language Studies* 16(1), 247–266. https://doi.org/10.1353/sls.1977.0019

Meier, R. (2006). The form of early signs: explaining signing children's articulatory development. In B. Schick, M. Marschark, & P. E. Spencer (Eds), *Advances in the sign language development of deaf children* (pp. 202–231). New York, NY: Oxford University Press.

Meier R. P., Cormier K., & Quinto-Pozos D. (2002). *Modality and structure in signed and spoken languages.* Cambridge: Cambridge University Press. https://doi.org/10.1017/CBO9780511486777

Meier, R. P., Mauk, C. E., Cheek, A., & Moreland, C. J. (2008). The form of children's early signs: Iconic or motoric determinants. *Language Learning & Development* 4(1), 63–98. https://doi.org/10.1080/15475440701377618

Morford, J. P. (2003). Grammatical development in adolescent first language learners. *Linguistics* 41(4), 681–721. https://doi.org/10.1515/ling.2003.022

Morford, J. P., & Carlson, M. L. (2011). Sign perception and recognition in non-native signers of ASL. *Language Learning & Development* 7(2), 149–168. https://doi.org/10.1080/15475441.2011.543393

Morgan, G., Barrett-Jones, S., & Stoneham, H. (2007). The first signs of language: Phonological development in British Sign Language. *Applied Psycholinguistics* 28, 3–22. https://doi.org/10.1017/S0142716407070014

Muir, L. J., & Richardson, I. E. (2005). Perception of sign language and its application to visual communications for deaf people. *Journal of Deaf Studies & Deaf Education* 10(4), 390–401. https://doi.org/10.1093/deafed/eni037

Newkirk, D., Klima, E., Pedersen, C. C., & Bellugi, U. (1980). Linguistic evidence from slips of the hand. In V. Fromkin (Ed.), *Errors in linguistic performance: slips of the tongue, ear, pen, and hand* (pp. 165–197). New York, NY: Academic Press.

Newport, E. L., & Meier, R. P. (1985). The acquisition of American Sign Language. In D. I. Slobin (Ed.), *The cross linguistic study of language acquisition, Volume 1: The data.* Hillsdale, NJ: Lawrence Erlbaum Associates.

Ortega, G. (2017). Iconicity and sign lexical acquisition: A review. *Frontiers in Psychology* 8, 1280. https://doi.org/10.3389/fpsyg.2017.01280

Ortega, G., & Morgan, G. (2015). Phonological development in hearing learners of a sign language: The role of sign complexity and iconicity. *Language Learning* 65(3), 660–668. https://doi.org/10.1111/lang.12123

Ortega, G., & Morgan, G. (2010). Comparing child and adult development of a visual phonological system. *Language Interaction & Acquisition* 1(1), 67–81. https://doi.org/10.1075/lia.1.1.05ort

Ortega, G., Sumer, B., & Ozyurek, A. (2017). Type of iconicity matters in the vocabulary development of signing children. *Developmental Psychology* 53(1), 89–99. https://doi.org/10.1037/dev0000161

Perniss, P., Lu, J. C., Morgan, G., & Vigliocco, G. (2018). Mapping language to the world: The role of iconicity in the sign language input. *Developmental Science* 21(2), e12551. https://doi.org/10.1111/desc.12551

Perniss, P., Thompson, R. L., & Vigliocco, G. (2010). Iconicity as a general property of language: Evidence from spoken and signed languages. *Frontiers in Psychology* 1, 227. https://doi.org/10.3389/fpsyg.2010.00227

Perry, L. K., Perlman, M., Winter, B., Massaro, D. W., & Lupyan, G. (2018). Iconicity in the speech of children and adults. *Developmental Science* 21(3), e12572. https://doi.org/10.1111/desc.12572

Petitto, L. A., & Marentette, P. (1991). Babbling in the manual mode: Evidence for the ontogeny of language. *Science* 251, 1483–1496. https://doi.org/10.1126/science.2006424

Pizer, G., Meier, R. P., & Shaw Points, K. (2011). Child-directed signing as a linguistic register. In R. Channon & H. van der Hulst (Eds.), *Formational units in sign languages* (pp. 65–86). Berlin: Walter de Gruyter. https://doi.org/10.1515/9781614510680.65

Reilly, J. S., McIntire, M. L., & Seago, H. (1992). Affective prosody in American Sign Language. *Sign Language Studies* 75, 113–128. https://doi.org/10.1353/sls.1992.0035

Ross, D. S., & Newport, E. L. (1996). The development of language from non-native linguistic input. In A. Stringfellow, D. Cahana-Amitay, E. Hughs, & A. Zukowski (Eds.), *Proceedings of the 20th annual Boston University Conference on Language Development* (volume 2, pp. 634–645). Somerville, MA: Cascadilla Press.

Sandler, W., & Lillo-Martin, D. (2006). *Sign language and linguistic universals*. Cambridge: Cambridge University Press. https://doi.org/10.1017/CBO9781139163910

Schick, B. (1990). The effects of morphosyntactic structure on the acquisition of classifier predicates in American Sign Language. In C. Lucas (Ed.), *Sign language research: Theoretical issues*. Washington, DC: Gallaudet University Press.

Schlenker, P. (2018). Visible meaning: Sign language and the foundations of semantics. *Theoretical Linguistics* 44(3–4): 123–208.

Shield, A., & Meier, R. P. (2018). Learning an embodied visual language: Four imitation strategies available to sign learners. *Frontiers in Psychology* 9, 811. https://doi.org/10.3389/fpsyg.2018.00811

Siedlecki, T., & Bonvillian, J. D. (1993). Location, handshape, and movement: Young children's acquisition of the formational aspects of American Sign Language. *Sign Language Studies* 78, 31–52. https://doi.org/10.1353/sls.1993.0016

Singleton, J. L., & Newport, E. L. (2004). When learners surpass their models: The acquisition of American Sign Language from inconsistent input. *Cognitive Psychology* 49(4), 370–407. https://doi.org/10.1016/j.cogpsych.2004.05.001

Siple, P. (1978). Visual constraints for sign language communication. *Sign Language Studies* 19, 95–110. https://doi.org/10.1353/sls.1978.0010

Smith, L. B., Quittner, A. L., Osberger, M. J., & Miyamoto R. (1998). Audition and visual attention: The developmental trajectory in deaf and hearing populations. *Developmental Psychology* 34(5), 840–850. https://doi.org/10.1037/0012-1649.34.5.840

Steinberg, L. (2005). Cognitive and affective development in adolescence. *Trends in Cognitive Sciences* 9(2), 69–74. https://doi.org/10.1016/j.tics.2004.12.005

Stoll, C., & Dye, M. W. G. (2019). Sign language experience redistributes attentional resources to the inferior visual field. *Cognition* 191, 103957. doi: https://doi.org/10.1016/j.cognition.2019.04.026

Stone, A., Petitto L., & Bosworth, R. (2018). Visual sonority modulates infants' attraction to sign language. *Language Learning & Development* 14(2), 130–148. https://doi.org/10.1080/15475441.2017.1404468

Swisher, M. V., Christie, K., & Miller, S. L. (1989). The reception of signs in peripheral vision by deaf persons. *Sign Language Studies* 63, 99–125. https://doi.org/10.1353/sls.1989.0011

Tharpe, A. M., Ashmead, D., Sladen, D. P., Ryan, H. A., & Rothpletz, A. M. (2008). Visual attention and hearing loss: Past and current perspectives. *Journal of the American Academy of Audiology* 19(10), 741–747. https://doi.org/10.3766/jaaa.19.10.2

Thompson, R. L. (2011). Iconicity in language processing and acquisition: What signed languages reveal. *Language & Linguistics Compass* 5, 603–616. https://doi.org/10.1111/j.1749-818X.2011.00301.x

Thompson, R. L, Emmorey, K., & Gollan, T. H. (2005). "Tip of the fingers" experiences by deaf signers. *Psychological Science* 16(11), 856–860. https://doi.org/10.1111/j.1467-9280.2005.01626.x

Thompson, R. L., Vinson, D. P., & Vigliocco, G. (2009). The link between form and meaning in American Sign Language: Lexical processing effects in a phonological decision task. *Journal of Experimental Psychology: Language, Memory, & Cognition* 35(2), 550–557.

Thompson, R. L., Vinson, D. P., Woll, B., & Vigliocco, G. (2012). The road to language learning is iconic: Evidence from British Sign Language. *Psychological Science* 23, 1443–1448. https://doi.org/10.1177/0956797612459763

Vinson, D. P., Thompson, R. L., Skinner, R., & Vigliocco, G. (2015). A faster path between meaning and form? Iconicity facilitates sign recognition and production in British Sign Language. *Journal of Memory & Language* 82, 56–85. https://doi.org/10.1016/j.jml.2015.03.002

Vinson, D. P., Thompson, R. L., Skinner, R., Fox, N., & Vigliocco, G. (2010). The hands and mouth do not always slip together in British Sign Language: Dissociating articulatory channels in the lexicon. *Psychological Science* 21(8), 1158–1167. https://doi.org/10.1177/0956797610377340

Watkins, F., & Thompson, R. L. (2017). The relationship between sign production and sign comprehension: What handedness reveals. *Cognition* 164, 144–149. https://doi.org/10.1016/j.cognition.2017.03.019

Waxman, S., Fu, X., Arunachalam, S., Leddon, E., Geraghty, K., & Song, H. J. (2013). Are nouns learned before verbs? Infants provide insight into a longstanding debate. *Child Development Perspectives* 7(3), 155–159. https://doi.org/10.1111/cdep.12032

Werker, J. F., & Tees, R. C. (1984). Cross-language speech perception: Evidence for perceptual reorganization during the first year of life. *Infant Behavioural Development* 7, 49–63. https://doi.org/10.1016/S0163-6383(84)80022-3

Woll, B. (1987). Historical and comparative aspects of BSL. In J. G. Kyle (Ed.), *Sign and school* (pp. 12–34). Clevedon: Multilingual Matters.

Woodward, J. C. (1976). Signs of change: historical variation in American Sign Language. *Sign Language Studies* 10, 81–94. https://doi.org/10.1353/sls.1976.0003

CHAPTER 9

Neurobiological insights from the study of deafness and sign language

Velia Cardin, Ruth Campbell, Mairéad MacSweeney,
Emil Holmer, Jerker Rönnberg and Mary Rudner

The study of deafness and sign language has provided a means of dissociating modality specificity from higher level abstract processes in the brain. Differentiating these is fundamental for establishing the relationship between sensorimotor representations and functional specialisation in the brain. Early deafness in humans provides a unique insight into this problem, because the reorganisation observed in the adult deaf brain is not only due to neural development in the absence of auditory inputs, but also due to the acquisition of visual communication strategies such as sign language and speechreading. Here we report research by scholars who have collaborated with Bencie Woll in understanding the neural reorganisation that occurs as a consequence of early deafness, and its relation to the use of different visual strategies for language. We concentrate on three main topics: functional specialisation of sensory cortices, language and working memory.

Introduction

For many people, the word language automatically means speech. It is perhaps not surprising that most of our knowledge of the neurobiology of language comes from the study of speech in hearing individuals. Similarly, our knowledge about perception derives mainly from studying the auditory cortex of hearing people or the visual cortex of sighted individuals. However, evidence obtained from exceptions to these rules has provided equally compelling yet unique insights into the capacities and limitations of the human brain.

Here, we discuss work that the authors have conducted together with Bencie Woll in the fields of sign language, speechreading and deafness, which we believe has contributed to our knowledge of language and cognition in the brain. Congenital deafness is an excellent model for the study of brain function

https://doi.org/10.1075/tilar.25.09car

and reorganisation, as adaptive changes develop not only in response to the lack of auditory stimulation, but also in response to visual mechanisms for language acquisition. This is because deaf individuals acquire language through the visual modality, and because language acquisition in deaf children is often delayed. Furthermore, because signed and spoken languages differ in regards to their underlying sensory and motor processes (sign languages are visual/manual languages, spoken languages are auditory/oral languages), they are excellent tools for investigating to what degree mental representations and processes are based on, or are independent of, underlying sensory and motor mechanisms. Focusing on neural plasticity, language and working memory, we discuss how neuroscience research on deafness has allowed us to better understand the effect of different developmental sensory and communication experiences on the structure and function of the adult brain.

Neural plasticity

Critical periods for the development of specific cognitive skills such as language have been proposed since the work of Lenneberg (1967; and see Chapter 6, Lillo-Martin, Smith & Tsimpli, this volume). Critical periods refer to time-limited periods in development when the acquisition of a cognitive skill may be achieved readily (or at all). This concept maps onto that of neural plasticity, which refers to the functional and structural capacity of the brain to reorganise in response to physiological or pathological environmental events (Merabet & Pascual-Leone, 2010). Neural events occurring at specific time points during development underlie such critical periods, and are mediated in the developing brain by enhanced cortical plasticity which allows the neural system to reorganise in response to environmental information (Hensch, 2004). In deaf individuals, one of the main causes of reorganisation is the absence of auditory inputs during a proposed critical period for development of the auditory system in the brain (Kral, 2013). However, there are other factors that drive plastic changes in the deaf brain, the most important ones being those related to the acquisition of language in the visual modality (Lyness et al., 2013). Because cortical plasticity varies as a function of sensory stimulation (and other environmental factors) during early sensitive periods (Lyness et al., 2013), we will only discuss studies of plasticity as a consequence of congenital or very early deafness. Individuals with late-acquired deafness or with cochlear implants may have access to auditory information during these critical periods, which will result in different developmental pathways for cortical regions involved in auditory and language processing (see section "*What are the consequences of impoverished access to early language?*").

The role of the "auditory" cortex in deaf individuals

Cortical auditory processing in hearing individuals is located largely in the Superior Temporal Cortex (STC). In some of the first neuroimaging studies in deaf individuals, it was shown that the STC of congenitally deaf humans responded to basic visual stimulation (moving dots; Finney et al., 2001), and to sign language (Nishimura et al., 1999). This "crossmodal plasticity" reflects the fact that regions typically involved in auditory processing can become responsive to other sensory inputs (Merabet & Pascual-Leone, 2010; Glick & Sharma, 2017). However, studying the effects of deafness on neural reorganisations is challenging because deafness has consequences beyond sensory processing, affecting cognitive skills including but not limited to language (see Dye & Thompson, Chapter 8 this volume). Given such heterogeneity, it is not surprising that in many studies of neural plasticity as a consequence of deafness, it is difficult to categorically establish if differences between hearing and deaf groups are due to differences in auditory experience, or due to delayed or poor language acquisition and skills.

In an effort to dissociate the effects of absence of auditory inputs during the critical periods from those of acquiring and using a signed or a spoken language, Cardin et al. (2013) conducted an fMRI experiment in which sign language stimuli were shown to three different groups of participants: (1) deaf native signers; (2) deaf non-signers – a group of individuals who were congenitally or early deaf, grew up using a spoken language, and did not know any sign language; and (3) hearing non-signers. The rationale of this study was that any plasticity effect that was due to a lack of auditory inputs during development will be present in both groups of deaf participants, but not in the group of hearing non-signers. On the other hand, given the linguistic content of the sign language stimuli, a plasticity effect as a consequence of early sign language acquisition will be found only in the group of deaf signers. The results showed that the absence of auditory inputs during infancy caused plasticity in the right posterior superior temporal cortex (STC – see Figure 1). Plasticity effects as a consequence of sign language use were found in both the left and right STC, and were evident only when stimuli had linguistic content. These regions recruited for sign language processing in deaf individuals corresponded to those supporting speech in hearing individuals. This suggests that in the absence of early sensory experience cortical regions develop their typical function, but adapt to a different type of sensory input, not only in terms of perception (Bennetti et al., 2017; Lomber et al., 2010), but also higher-order cognitive function. As we discuss in the section below, it is indeed the case that regions involved in spoken language processing in hearing individuals maintain their specific role, at least to some extent, in phonological, semantic and syntactic processing in deaf individuals, either for speechreading (lipreading) or sign language (Corina and Knapp, 2006; MacSweeney et al., 2008a; Campbell and Macsweeney, 2012; Twomey et al., 2017).

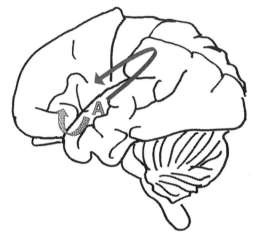

Figure 1. Schematic of left hemisphere lateral surface showing perisylvian regions centred on 'A', (secondary) auditory cortex in the superior temporal lobe (STC – see text). The dark arrow indicates the dorsal projection stream and the stippled arrow the approximate route of the ventral projection – both to inferior frontal regions.

The types of stimuli and tasks that reveal plasticity effects in the STC suggest an involvement of this region in higher order sensory processing. This is supported by studies that used other brain imaging techniques such as EEG and MEG to investigate the timing of this response. In a MEG study, Leonard et al. (2012) showed that responses to sign language (and static pictures) arose from the STC of deaf individuals during a late time window (~ 300 ms) associated to lexicosemantic processing. Early sensory processing responses (~ 100 ms) were constrained to visual cortices in both hearing and deaf adults. (For a further example see Bottari et al., 2014). The next step for understanding the role of the superior temporal regions in deaf individuals is to go beyond language and low-level vision, and investigate other cognitive functions. In the past few years, studies have shown that the STC is involved in visual working memory (Buchsbaum et al., 2005; Cardin et al., 2018; Ding et al., 2015). This effect is independent both of the linguistic content of the stimuli, and of the language knowledge of the deaf participants, which indicates that it is not directly related to language processing in the STC (Cardin et al., 2018). Instead, it suggests a different role for some regions of the STC in deaf individuals – a role which is distinct from the one this cortical region has in hearing individuals. Analogous functional changes have been reported in the visual cortex of blind individuals (Röder et al., 2002; Amedi et al., 2004; Bedny et al., 2015). These functional changes suggest considerable malleability in the function of brain regions that are usually considered unisensory, and the function of such regions in the adult brain will strongly depend on the type and quality of early environmental experience. Together, these findings point to two co-existing plasticity mechanisms: functional preservation and functional change. Future efforts should be directed towards delineating the physiological and anatomical principles behind each of them.

Modality dependent and independent language networks

Visual speech in deaf and hearing individuals

The movement of the speech articulators can be felt by the speaker, and is seen as well as heard. Sensitivity to seen speech can be demonstrated from the first months of life in hearing infants (e.g. Dodd, 1980; Mercure et al., 2018) and, while audition dominates, speech processing continues to be essentially multimodal throughout life (Campbell, 2008). Behavioral studies show that seeing the speaker enhances the perception of heard speech – especially, but not exclusively, when speech is noisy (Dodd & Campbell, 1988).

It might be assumed that deaf children, denied access to heard language, must become efficient speechreaders. However, younger deaf children can be worse speechreaders than hearing children (Kyle et al., 2013), although deaf adults often outperform hearing people on tests of speechreading (Mohammed et al., 2006). It is likely that skilled speechreading in deaf adults makes use of multiple strategies to infer the meaning of the speechread message (Feld & Sommers, 2009); and see section on working memory below. Skilled speechreading is effortful, and it can make greater demands on general cognitive processes than hearing speech (e.g., Hornsby, 2013). The hearing speechreader has less need to develop these skills, which could explain the difference in performance in the adult populations.

Many speech actions are hidden within the mouth, leading to suboptimal identification of phonemes by sight alone. That does not necessarily mean that speechreading is ineffective as a route into language for someone who cannot hear, but its utility varies not just with the content of speech and its general visibility, but also with the language experience of the speechreader. For instance, knowledge of the statistical structure of words in the language can often make up for the lack of phonological detail (Auer and Bernstein, 1997). There can be a good deal of variability in speechreading skill in deaf people, reflecting, amongst other factors, their varied exposure to and affiliation with spoken language. A partial analogue, for hearing people, would be the ability to interpret noisy or degraded speech: that too shows marked individual variation (Rönnberg et al., 2013; Tamati et al., 2013).

Neural bases of audiovisual speech processing in hearing individuals

Neural models of speech processing in hearing adults can provide a template against which to explore speechreading in hearing and deaf populations. These models differ in several regards, but they propose that in order to extract a linguistic message, speech processing is supported by a network of left-lateralised perisylvian regions (Figure 1). Sounds reaching the primary auditory cortex in Heschl's gyrus within the superior temporal plane (hidden from view in the surface representation of Figure 1) are then processed in the STC. Activation in the STC maps, via connection tracts, onto regions in the inferior frontal gyrus (IFG) which are specialised for articulatory processing (a 'dorsal route'). This route is thought to effect the processing of speech structure, including phonology. A complementary route for the processing of semantic speech-based entities maps from the anterior STC to inferior frontal regions (Hickok & Poeppel, 2007; Rauschecker & Scott, 2009 – a 'ventral route', and see previous section). The left-lateralization of all these processes is age-dependent, and evidence of left-lateralization for speech processing is less secure in children than adults (Neville & Bavelier, 1998; Holland et al., 2007).

Neuroscientific studies of audiovisual speech processing have shown that perisylvian auditory speech regions are also activated by seen speech (Calvert et al., 1997). These activations in the STC seem to follow a modality gradient: auditory speech preferentially activates more anterior regions, visual speech (speechreading) more posterior regions, while mid-regions of the sulcus preferentially specialize for audiovisual speech processing (Bernstein & Liebenthal, 2014; Venezia et al., 2017). In accordance to this gradient, more anterior regions of the STS show greater activation for speech and language processing (Beauchamp, 2015; Deen et al., 2015), whereas more posterior parts of the STS show greater activation for bodily and facial gestures (non-verbal signals; see Figure 2). In addition, visual perception of nonverbal biological signals, such as those seen when someone speaks, also engages regions specialized for the perception of face actions and biological movement in the parieto-temporo-occipital junction region (Calvert and Campbell, 2003).

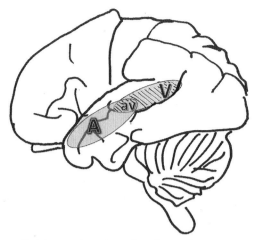

Figure 2. Schematic of left hemisphere lateral surface indicating approximate regions within superior temporal cortex specialized for auditory processing of speech (A: open region) and visual gesture processing (V: stippled region). Regions specialized for auditory-visual processing of speech are in the mid regions of these superior temporal structures, with projections from both auditory and visual processing.

Neural bases for speechreading in deaf people

Given these findings in hearing people, how might seen speech localise in the brains of deaf people? Would we expect to find evidence of more extensive – or different – patterns of activation? Might the brains of deaf people show greater activation in 'purely' visual regions than those of hearing people, since deaf people rely more on speechreading?

One study (Capek et al., 2008a), compared deaf and hearing adults on a simple speechreading task (identifying a videoclip of a spoken word 'yes' by sight among other silently spoken unconnected words). The deaf participants showed more extensive activation than the hearing group in the left STC, specifically. Ludman et al. (2000) previously showed that speechreading skill in hearing people correlated specifically with activation in the STC, so this difference between groups could reflect differences in speechreading skill, which was better for the deaf participants. Activations in the anterior STC did correlate with speechreading skill in both deaf and hearing people (Capek et al., 2008a). However, the differences between groups persisted when speechreading skill was controlled. This finding, then, suggests that when hearing is absent, anterior parts of the left STC that process heard speech in hearing people can 'take over' speechreading.

Speech actions in sign language and in seen speech: Neural correlates

The deaf participants in the Capek et al. (2008a,b) study were all bimodal bilingual – that is, they were similarly proficient in both BSL and speechreading. Could the more extensive left STC activation observed for speechreading in these deaf people simply reflect their bimodal language skills? This particular study formed part of a set of explorations of perception of mouth actions in both sign language and speech. Sign languages incorporate mouth actions alongside manual ones, and their role has been explored by sign linguists (Baker & Padden, 1978; Sutton-Spence & Woll, 1999). The comparison of activation patterns for seen speech compared with mouth actions in BSL that were not speechlike re-iterated and extended the previous finding: speechreading activated more anterior parts of the STC, while BSL non-speechlike mouth actions activated more posterior parts (Capek et al., 2008a, 2010). When these bimodal bilingual deaf adults were compared to hearing adults born into signing families (hearing bimodal bilinguals), deafness itself was found to have an influence on the pattern: once again, deaf speechreaders showed greater activation in anterior parts of the STC than did bilingual hearing people (Capek et al., 2008b).

Taken together, these findings suggest that early developmental experience modulates functional specialization in the STC. These regions appear to show plasticity reflecting both early auditory experiences *and* language processing. In this respect the findings for speechreading recapitulate those described previously, in the section on sign language processing. However, the cortical regions that show plasticity may differ depending on the nature of the visual language signal. Plasticity for speechreading in the brains of deaf individuals is seen in the anterior STC (Capek et al., 2008a) – those regions that are regularly activated by heard speech in hearing people. By contrast, sign language plasticity is seen in more posterior regions, specialized for visual processing, where deaf people show greater activation than hearing people (Cardin et al., 2013, 2016).

Sign languages as a window into modality-independent language processing

Studies with native users of a signed language provide a unique opportunity to identify the neural systems supporting higher order language acquisition and processing *regardless of modality*. Identification of regions of overlapping activation during tasks performed in signed and spoken languages allows us to directly test the hypothesis that these regions are involved in language development and processing independently of modality. Here we review neural systems which are recruited by native adult users of sign language (studies with children are lacking at present).

In accordance with lesion studies of hearing patients, studies of native signers with lesions overwhelmingly indicate that left hemisphere damage leads to severely impaired language processing (aphasia) while right hemisphere damage does not (e.g. Hickok et al., 1996; Marshall et al., 2005). Neuroimaging studies also indicate a critical role for the left hemisphere in sign language processing. Despite differences in the articulators used to produce sign and speech, both modalities of language production predominantly engage left hemisphere regions (Emmorey et al., 2014; Gutierrez-Sigut et al., 2015, 2016). With regard to language *perception*, a left fronto-temporal network involving the superior temporal gyrus and sulcus (STC) as well as the left inferior frontal gyrus, extending into the prefrontal gyrus, was shown to be involved in processing both sign and speech (see also Sakai et al., 2005). Numerous studies have also identified a primarily left lateralized fronto-temporal network involved in sign language perception when contrasted with gesture (Newman et al., 2015), transitive actions (Corina et al., 2007) or non-sense movement (MacSweeney et al., 2004). These studies suggest that the core left-lateralized language network is resilient to change in language modality. In summary, even though language development in native users of signed and spoken languages involves different sensorimotor mechanisms, very similar left-perisylvian networks are engaged for the perception and production of sign and speech. This similarity appears to extend to metalinguistic judgments regarding the sublexical, phonological, structure of sign and speech, which have been shown to engage a left fronto-parietal network (MacSweeney et al., 2008b).

Although the overlap between the networks supporting sign and speech processing is extensive, there are some differences. As indicated in previous parts of this chapter, direct contrasts have highlighted differences reflecting early sensory processing. Audio-visual speech elicits greater activation than sign language in auditory processing regions in the STC. In contrast, signed languages elicit greater activation than audio-visual speech in biological motion processing regions of the posterior middle temporal gyri, bilaterally (Emmorey et al., 2014; Söderfeldt et al., 1997; MacSweeney et al., 2002b). Above and beyond sensory demands of visual motion processing, the posterior middle temporal gyri also appear to be recruited when visual movement is specifically linguistic, such as in the perception of classifiers representing movement of a referent (MacSweeney et al., 2002a; McCullough et al., 2012).

There is also growing evidence suggesting that the left inferior and superior parietal lobules play a greater role in sign language processing than spoken language processing (see MacSweeney et al., 2008a for review). It has been suggested that the left superior parietal lobule may be involved in motor rehearsal during memory tasks (Buchsbaum et al., 2005) and/or in proprioceptive monitoring during sign production (Emmorey et al., 2016). Within the inferior parietal lobule

(IPL), the left supramarginal gyrus appears to play a particularly important role in phonological processing of signed language (Corina et al., 1999; MacSweeney et al., 2008b; Cardin et al., 2016).

The summary of the literature regarding signed and spoken language processing presented above refers to both deaf and hearing signers. It is worth noting that, in addition to the networks described above, deaf signers appear to recruit parts of the STC that are not activated in hearing sign users (MacSweeney et al., 2002b; Cardin et al., 2016; Twomey et al., 2017). As described in the section on plasticity, the STCs are involved in auditory processing in the hearing. In congenitally deaf participants, these regions are available to process input from other modalities. Of particular relevance to this section, posterior parts of the left STC in deaf signers appear to be particularly sensitive to the demands of sign language processing and not to general low-level visuo-spatial processing demands (Cardin et al., 2013; Twomey et al., 2017). It is unlikely that this effect is language specific, but rather due to the complexity the visual components of the language and the potential increased processing demands. However, further studies are necessary to explore this hypothesis directly.

What are the neural consequences of impoverished access to early language?

All of the studies reviewed above have focused on studies of deaf native signers. However, the vast majority of deaf children are not exposed to a signed language from birth. They are born to hearing non-signing parents, who may or may not decide to learn a signed language. Often these children are exposed to a signed language at school or upon leaving school, at an age past the point that would normally be considered the critical period for language development (see Mayberry & Lock, 2003; Mayberry, Lock, & Kazmi, 2002). These children have extremely heterogeneous language experiences and can provide unique insights into the influence of timing on the development of the language system.

Although the impact of late sign language acquisition on sign language processing has been investigated extensively at the behavioral level (see Lillo-Martin, et al, this volume), the impact of late sign language acquisition on the neural systems supporting language has yet to be fully explored. Hearing late learners of sign have already successfully acquired a first (spoken) language; deaf late learners of a signed language have not. When a deaf person learns a sign language later in life, it is typically built on impoverished early access to a spoken language. That is, it cannot always be considered a second language, as is clearly the case for hearing late learners of a signed language.

To date only a handful of studies have examined the impact of late sign language acquisition on the neural systems supporting sign language processing in those born deaf. MacSweeney et al. (2008b) tested deaf native and non-native signers. Participants were asked to make phonological judgements about signs (same location?) and speech (rhyme?) in response to picture pairs. Increased activations were found in the left inferior frontal gyrus in the non-native compared to the native signers (MacSweeney et al., 2008a). Critically, this was the case not only for the task in BSL, which was learnt late, but also for the task in English, of which both groups had similar experience and had also shown equal levels of performance on English online (rhyme task) and offline tasks. One interpretation of these data is that having a robust first language (here a signed language) provides a solid basis upon which to learn a second language (here English). These data support behavioral data underlining the critical importance of early language experience, in any modality, for later language development (Mayberry et al., 2002).

Mayberry et al. (2011; see also Lillo-Martin et al., this volume) also investigated the influence of age of sign language acquisition by testing participants whose age of onset of American Sign Language (ASL) acquisition ranged from birth to 14 years old. Participants were tested on phonemic and grammatical judgements in response to ASL sentences. In contrast to the findings of MacSweeney et al. (2008b), Mayberry et al. (2011) found *decreased* recruitment of left frontal regions in late compared to early signers. Late signers showed enhanced recruitment of occipital cortices. There were a number of stimulus (ASL video / static pictures) and task differences between the MacSweeney et al. (2008b) and Mayberry et al. (2011) studies that may have contributed to the different pattern of results. One key difference is that the participants in the MacSweeney et al. (2008b) study are likely to have had better spoken language skills than those in the Mayberry et al. (2011) study. Whatever the cause for the difference in results between these two studies, it is clear that the left inferior frontal cortices are sensitive (in one direction or another) to the age of sign language acquisition and/or to the consequences of impoverished first language input. Future studies are needed to dissociate effects that are related to age of sign language exposure and those related to sign language proficiency.

Mayberry and colleagues have also had the opportunity to examine ASL processing in two deaf adolescents who moved to the US from Central America and who are described as having no first language (spoken language) before encountering ASL at the age of 14 years (Ferjan Ramirez et al., 2014). Critically, only in cases of extreme deprivation could such cases be found in the hearing population. These case studies therefore offer unique insights into the consequences of severe early language deprivation. Using MEG the authors showed that even after three years of exposure to ASL, the teenager's responses to single signs were highly atypical, engaging right dorsal fronto-parietal regions, rather than the typical left-lateralized fronto-temporal network (Ferjan Ramirez et al., 2016). When followed up just over a year later, these cases still showed atypical neural processing for less familiar signs. However, interestingly, for more familiar signs they started to show activation in the typical left perisylvian network. The authors argue that even though timing of language experience inevitably affects the organization of neural language processing, language representation in the human brain can continue to evolve with experience, even into adolescence (Ferjan Ramirez et al., 2016). Continuing to study the language development of these individuals and testing them on more complex language input will provide unique insights into the consequences of extremely impoverished early language experience on the neural bases of language processing.

Working memory for language in deaf and hearing individuals

The general notion of a working memory is that of a limited-capacity mental work-bench that allows for storage and manipulation of information (Baddeley & Hitch, 1974; Daneman & Merikle, 1996). Although working memory is in place already in infancy (Zosh & Feigenson, 2015), it develops steadily during childhood (Cowan, 2016), and it represents one of the most central cognitive functions in the adult brain. Furthermore, there is a well-supported proposal that the development of working memory and the acquisition of native phonology and first words are closely and reciprocally linked (Gathercole & Baddeley, 1993). How this plays out in relation to language processing in deaf children and adults is the topic of this section which reviews studies of working memory for sign and spoken language.

Linguistic representations and working memory development

Due to its relevance for cognitive models of working memory (Baddeley & Hitch, 1974; Rönnberg et al., 2013; Rönnberg et al., 2018), many efforts have concentrated on understanding the role of phonological representations during working memory for sign language. According to the Ease of Language Understanding model (ELU, Rönnberg et al., 2013; Rönnberg, Holmer & Rudner, 2019), lexical access (irrespective of language modality) is mediated by phonological representations that "unlock" the lexical/semantic meaning. Whether there is an actual match in the number of phonological and semantic attributes is assumed to be set by a threshold. Below threshold, lexical access is denied. In this case, a mismatch is said to have occurred (Rudner et al., 2009; Rönnberg et al., 2013). Considering the importance of phonological matching during speech processing, a role for phonology during sign language processing may be expected. While speech phonology is based on sound patterns generated through the vocal tract, sign phonology is mainly based on the articulatory patterns of the moving hands in terms of shape, position, movement and orientation. Work by Wilson and Emmorey (1997) using ASL provided evidence for a sign version of the phonological loop (Baddeley, 2012). We have reported evidence of a phonological similarity effect for Swedish Sign Language (SSL, Rudner & Rönnberg, 2008; Andin et al., 2013) although we did not find such an effect in BSL (Andin et al., 2013), possibly due to methodological differences. Subsequent work shows that phonological representations play a less prominent role in working memory for sign language than is suggested by generic models of working memory (Rudner et al., 2016; Rudner, 2018; Rudner and Rönnberg, 2019). Rather, it is the nature of the underlying motor representations that is important for explicit processing of signs (Rudner, 2015; Cardin et al., 2016; Rudner et al., 2016), in line with the notion of embodied cognition (Wilson, 2001; Rönnberg et al., 2004)

Holmer et al. (2016) investigated the role of sign-phonology representations for sign language working memory in the developing cognitive system. In their study, Holmer et al. (2016) found that requiring children to imitate (lists of) manual gestures improved performance more for deaf and hard-of-hearing signing children than for hearing non-signing children. For successful imitation to occur, representations must be kept in mind before a judgement can be passed, which means that the ability to imitate is dependent on working memory. Thus, the steeper development in the hard-of-hearing signing children than the hearing non-signing children reported by Holmer et al. (2016) is likely to reflect a supportive role of existing phonological representations of signs in developing working memory for signs. On a similar note, Pierce et al. (2017) argued that the role of early language experience in establishing linguistic representations is crucial for the development of phonological working memory. In addition, they proposed that the state of phonological working memory at any given time will constrain further learning.

However, linguistic representations seem not only to influence the development of working memory for linguistic material but also non-linguistic working memory. In a study by Marshall et al. (2015), individual differences in non-linguistic working memory was in part explained by level of vocabulary in a group of deaf signing children. In a later study, Botting et al. (2017) reported that language skills mediated executive functioning skill, including working memory. Experiences that prepare the brain for language processing, by establishment of linguistic representations, are also important for the emerging working memory system in the brain.

Modality-specific and modality-independent working memory mechanisms

Working memory seen from a communicative perspective is assumed to serve both predictive and postdictive linguistic functions (Rönnberg et al., 2019). The predictive function is related to the ability to maintain focus while, for example, inhibiting distracting information (Sörqvist & Rönnberg, 2012) or improving recognition by means of phonological or semantic priming (Signoret et al., 2018). The postdictive aspect is about reconstructing and repairing what has been missed or misperceived in a more elaborative way than for prediction. Here, rehearsal of elements of the dialogue, combined with retrieval from semantic long-term memory may be used to infer the missing information (Rönnberg et al., 2013).

Within this framework, the study of working memory for sign language and speech allow us to understand what aspects of working memory in a communication setting are due to the specific sensorimotor mechanisms used for perception and production of the language (modality specific), and what aspects are shared across language modalities, potentially based on higher level linguistic representations (modality-independent).

In a study of working memory for sign and speech in bimodal bilingual hearing individuals, Rönnberg et al. (2004) demonstrated that working memory for signs and speech obey similar laws of memory. In terms of an analysis of serial position effects, typical bow-shaped curves were obtained, demonstrating both recency and pre-recency effects, with an overall superiority for spoken tokens. A subset of *early*, hearing native bilinguals even showed that the effect of language modality was non-significant. Thus, this result means that there are modality-independent commonalities across linguistic modalities.

Nevertheless, imaging data from studies of working memory for sign language, both in deaf and hearing individuals, showed language modality-specific bilateral parietal and occipital activations for the contrast of signs over speech (Rönnberg et al., 2004; Rudner et al., 2007; Pa et al., 2009). These differences could be explained by activation differences in sensorimotor cortex elicited by the two different types of stimuli – signs will result in activations in parietooccipital regions, whereas speech will result in activations in temporal areas. To test whether parieto-occipital activations during working memory for sign language were due to modality-specific linguistic processing or sensorimotor processing, we conducted an experiment in which we compared working memory for lexical signs and working memory for nonsense moving objects in groups of deaf and hearing participants with and without knowledge of sign language (Cardin et al., 2018). Crucially, we used point-light stimuli, significantly reducing the differences in low-level features between the stimuli. Our results showed no specific activation for working memory for signs compared with nonsense objects, suggesting that differences in working memory for linguistic and non-linguistic visual stimuli identified in previous less well-controlled studies were driven by activations in areas involved in sensorimotor processing of the stimuli, which could also be involved in storing information during working memory tasks.

In spite of this, there is a possibility that it is the type of processing (or mechanism involved in the particular processing invoked) that is crucial for language modality specific effects to occur, and not necessarily the types of stimuli used. For example, Rudner et al. (2007) investigated the episodic buffer of working memory in bimodal bilinguals using n-back lists. The task requires that subjects keep track of the sequence of events (signs/words) in order to retrieve one event that may match another one presented earlier – just how many steps back varied from trial to trial (hence 'n-back'). The critical (mixed) list contained both lexical signs and spoken words to be compared across modality/language. These mixed lists demanded deep semantic analysis, a kind of binding process in the episodic buffer of working memory between the lexical meaning of signs and words. Compared to unimodal lists, the mixed list data produced activity in right middle temporal brain areas. This may indicate that there is a neural correlate of the episodic buffer that actually connects signs with speech by binding phonological representations in the speech and sign loops of working memory to semantic memory representations in long-term memory (Rudner et al., 2007). Furthermore, using an n-back task, Rudner et al. (2013) also showed language-modality specific effects at different levels of processing stimuli (semantic, phonological and orthographic).

The overall picture that arises from these working memory studies is that language modality specificity seems to lie in the type of mental operations induced rather in the sensory input as such (Wilson & Emmorey, 1997). What type of operation within working memory is actually asked for (e.g., semantic judgements, serial recall, phonological comparisons, same/different judgments) appears to be the main determinant of brain signatures.

Conclusion

Bencie Woll's pioneering and ongoing studies into sign language processes have allowed us, as her colleagues and collaborators, to develop a variety of insights into the impact of deafness and sign language exposure on the development of functional specialisations in the adult brain. Sign language studies of language and working memory processing have shown largely modality-independent mechanisms. These are used for general-purpose processing, independently of the sensorimotor properties of the stimuli, and ultimately challenge theories based on sensorimotor properties of specific signals. Furthermore, neuroscience research on deafness and sign language has provided unique information about the potential of the brain for change throughout development, including infancy (when the roots of language are laid down). It is clear that neural plasticity effects can be observed as a consequence of deafness, both in auditory and non-auditory cortices, and that deafness as a model allows a much fuller interpretation of the plastic possibilities of the adult brain. Evidence from the study of deafness shows that regions considered to be dedicated to specific sensory and articulatory processes are also activated by inputs and outputs from another modality. In addition, the study of the brain in deaf individuals has clarified the function(s) of those modality-independent networks which support language processing, whether signed or spoken. However, a bigger issue is still pending – what is the functional and behavioural relevance of the reorganisation observed in the brain of deaf individuals? In animal models, a causal relationship has been established between enhanced performance in specific visual tasks and crossmodal plasticity in the auditory cortex. In humans, plastic reorganisation as a consequence of deafness also seems to impact behaviour (Bottari et al., 2011; Karns et al., 2012; Ding et al., 2015), but we are far from understanding the all-encompassing implications of these effects and the principles governing them. Altogether, the study of deafness and sign language have allowed us to gain a better understanding of the developmental adaptability of the neural system and its largely modality-independent processes.

References

Amedi, A., Floel, A., Knecht, S., Zohary, E., & Cohen, L. G. (2004). Transcranial magnetic stimulation of the occipital pole interferes with verbal processing in blind subjects. *Nat. Neurosci.*, 7, 1266–1270.

Andin J., Orfanidou, E., Cardin, V., Holmer, E., Capek, C. M., Woll, B., Rönnberg, J., & Rudner, M. (2013). Similar digit-based working memory in deaf signers and hearing non-signers despite digit span differences. *Front. Psychol.*, 4, 942. Available at: <http://www.pubmed-central.nih.gov/articlerender.fcgi?artid=3863759&tool=pmcentrez&rendertype=abstract>

Auer, E. T., & Bernstein, L. E. (1997) Speechreading and the structure of the lexicon: Computationally modeling the effects of reduced phonetic distinctiveness on lexical uniqueness. *J. Acoust. Soc. Am.*, 102, 3704–3710. Available at: <http://www.ncbi.nlm.nih.gov/pubmed/9407662> (Accessed 14 October, 2017).

Baddeley, A. (2012). Working memory: Theories, models, and controversies. *Annu. Rev. Psychol.*, 63, 1–29 Available at: <www.annualreviews.org> (Accessed 14 October, 2017).

Baddeley, A. D., & Hitch, G. (1974). Working memory. *Psychology of Learning and Motivation*, 8, 47–89 Available at: <http://linkinghub.elsevier.com/retrieve/pii/S0079742108604521> (Accessed 3 October, 2017).

Baker C., & Padden, C. (1978). Focussing on the non-manual components of ASL. In P. Siple (Ed.), *Understanding language through sign language research* (pp. 27–57). New York, NY: Academic Press.

Beauchamp, M. S. (2015). The social mysteries of the superior temporal sulcus. *Trends Cogn. Sci.*, 19, 489–490 Available at: <http://linkinghub.elsevier.com/retrieve/pii/S1364661315001539> (Accessed 4 October, 2017).

Bedny, M., Richardson, H., & Saxe, R. (2015). "Visual" cortex responds to spoken language in blind children. *J. Neurosci.*, 35, 11674–11681.

Bernstein, L. E., & Liebenthal, E. (2014). Neural pathways for visual speech perception. *Front. Neurosci.*, 8, 386. Available at: <http://www.ncbi.nlm.nih.gov/pubmed/25520611> (Accessed 4 October, 2017).

Bottari, D., Caclin, A., Giard, M.-H., & Pavani, F. (2011). Changes in early cortical visual processing predict enhanced reactivity in deaf individuals. *PLoS One, 6:e25607* Available at: <http://www.pubmedcentral.nih.gov/articlerender.fcgi?artid=3183070&tool=pmcentrez&rendertype=abstract> (Accessed 11 June, 2015).

Bottari, D., Heimler, B., Caclin, A., Dalmolin, A., Giard, M.-H., & Pavani, F. (2014). Visual change detection recruits auditory cortices in early deafness. *Neuroimage*, 94, 172–184 Available at: <http://www.ncbi.nlm.nih.gov/pubmed/24636881>

Botting, N., Jones, A., Marshall, C., Denmark, T., Atkinson, J., & Morgan, G. (2017). Non-verbal executive function is mediated by language: A study of deaf and hearing children. *Child Dev.*, 88, 1689–1700.

Buchsbaum, B., Pickell, B., Love, T., Hatrak, M., Bellugi, U., & Hickok, G. (2005). Neural substrates for verbal working memory in deaf signers: fMRI study and lesion case report. *Brain Lang.*, 95, 265–272. Available at: <http://www.ncbi.nlm.nih.gov/pubmed/16246734> (Accessed 20 June, 2014).

Calvert, G. A., Bullmore, E., Brammer, M., Campbell, R., Williams, S., McGuire, P., & David, A. (1997). Activation of auditory cortex during silent lipreading. *Science*, 276, 593–596. doi: https://doi.org/10.1126/science.276.5312.593

Calvert, G. A., & Campbell, R. (2003). Reading speech from still and moving faces: The neural substrates of visible speech. *J. Cogn. Neurosci.*, 15, 57–70 Available at: <http://www.ncbi.nlm.nih.gov/pubmed/12590843> (Accessed 31 October, 2018).

Campbell, R. (2008). The processing of audio-visual speech: Empirical and neural bases. *Philos. Trans. R. Soc. L. B. Biol. Sci.*, 363,1001–1010.

Campbell, R., & Macsweeney, M. (2012). Brain bases for seeing speech: FMRI studies of speechreading. In G. Bailly, P. Perrier, & E. Vatikiotis-Bateson (Eds.), Audiovisual speech processing (pp. 76–100). Cambridge: Cambridge University Press. Available at: <http://discovery.ucl.ac.uk/1407709/> (Accessed 11 June, 2015).

Capek, C. M., Macsweeney, M., Woll, B., Waters, D., McGuire, P. K., David, A. S., Brammer, M. J., & Campbell, R. (2008a). Cortical circuits for silent speechreading in deaf and hearing people. *Neuropsychologia*, 46, 1233–1241. Available at: <http://www.ncbi.nlm.nih.gov/pubmed/18249420>

Capek, C. M., Waters, D., Woll, B., MacSweeney, M., Brammer, M. J., McGuire, P. K., David, A. S., & Campbell, R. (2008b). Hand and mouth: Cortical correlates of lexical processing in British Sign Language and speechreading English. *J. Cogn. Neurosci.*, 20, 1220–1234. Available at: <http://www.pubmedcentral.nih.gov/articlerender.fcgi?artid=3370423&tool=pmcentrez&rendertype=abstract>

Capek, C. M., Woll, B., MacSweeney, M., Waters, D., McGuire, P. K., David, A. S., Brammer, M. J., & Campbell, R. (2010). Superior temporal activation as a function of linguistic knowledge: Insights from deaf native signers who speechread. *Brain Lang.*, 112, 129–134. Available at: <http://www.pubmedcentral.nih.gov/articlerender.fcgi?artid=3398390&tool=pmcentrez&rendertype=abstract> (Accessed 20 June, 2014).

Cardin, V., Orfanidou, E., Kästner, L., Rönnberg, J., Woll, B., Capek, C. M., & Rudner, M. (2016). Monitoring different phonological parameters of sign language engages the same cortical language network but distinctive perceptual ones. *J. Cogn. Neurosci.*, 28, 20–40. Available at: <http://www.ncbi.nlm.nih.gov/pubmed/26351993> (Accessed 11 August, 2016).

Cardin, V., Orfanidou, E., Rönnberg, J., Capek, C. M., Rudner, M., & Woll, B. (2013). Dissociating cognitive and sensory neural plasticity in human superior temporal cortex. *Nat. Commun.*, 4, 1473. Available at: <http://www.nature.com/doifinder/10.1038/ncomms2463>

Cardin, V., Rudner, M., De Oliveira, R. F., Andin, J. T., Su, M., Beese, L., Woll, B., & Rönnberg, J. (2018) The organization of working memory networks is shaped by early sensory experience. *Cereb. Cortex*, 28, 3540–3355. Available at: <http://academic.oup.com/cercor/article/doi/10.1093/cercor/bhx222/4097584/The-Organization-of-Working-Memory-Networks-is> (Accessed 3 October, 2017).

Corina, D., Chiu, Y.-S., Knapp, H., Greenwald, R., San Jose-Robertson, L., & Braun, A. (2007). Neural correlates of human action observation in hearing and deaf subjects. *Brain Res.*, 1152, 111–129. Available at: <http://www.ncbi.nlm.nih.gov/pubmed/17459349> (Accessed 31 October, 2018).

Corina, D., & Knapp, H. (2006). Sign language processing and the mirror neuron system. *Cortex*, 42, 529–539. Available at: <http://www.sciencedirect.com/science/article/pii/S0010945208703939> (Accessed 27 June, 2014).

Corina, D. P., McBurney, S. L., Dodrill, C., Hinshaw, K., Brinkley, J., & Ojemann, G. (1999). Functional roles of Broca's area and SMG: Evidence from cortical stimulation mapping in a deaf signer. *Neuroimage*, 10, 570–581. Available at: <http://www.ncbi.nlm.nih.gov/pubmed/10547334> (Accessed 17 July, 2014).

Cowan, N. (2016). Working memory maturation: Can we get at the essence of cognitive growth? *Perspect. Psychol. Sci.*, 11, 239–264. Available at: <http://journals.sagepub.com/doi/10.1177/1745691615621279> (Accessed 31 October, 2018).

Daneman, M., & Merikle, P. M. (1996). Working memory and language comprehension: A meta-analysis. *Psychon. Bull. Rev.*, 3, 422–433. Available at: <http://www.springerlink.com/index/10.3758/BF03214546> (Accessed 3 October, 2017).

Deen, B., Koldewyn, K., Kanwisher, N., & Saxe, R. (2015). Functional organization of social perception and cognition in the superior temporal sulcus. *Cereb. Cortex*, 25, 4596–4609. Available at: <http://www.ncbi.nlm.nih.gov/pubmed/26048954> (Accessed 4 October, 2017).

Ding, H., Qin, W., Liang, M., Ming, D., Wan, B., Li, Q., Yu, C. (2015). Cross-modal activation of auditory regions during visuo-spatial working memory in early deafness. *Brain*, 138, 2750–2765. Available at: <http://www.ncbi.nlm.nih.gov/pubmed/26070981> (Accessed 7 October, 2015).

Dodd, B. (1980). Interaction of auditory and visual information in speech perception. *Br. J. Psychol.*, 71, 541–549. Available at: <http://www.ncbi.nlm.nih.gov/pubmed/7437675> (Accessed 1 November, 2018).

Dodd, B., & Campbell, R. (1988). Hearing by eye: The psychology of lip-reading. *Am. J. Psychol.*, 101, 598. Available at: <http://www.jstor.org/stable/1423237?origin=crossref> (Accessed 4 October, 2017).

Emmorey, K., McCullough, S., Mehta, S., Grabowski, T. J. (2014). How sensory-motor systems impact the neural organization for language: Direct contrasts between spoken and signed language. *Front. Psychol.*, 5, 484. Available at: <http://www.ncbi.nlm.nih.gov/pubmed/24904497> (Accessed 9 August, 2016).

Emmorey, K., McCullough, S., & Weisberg, J. (2016). The neural underpinnings of reading skill in deaf adults. *Brain Lang.*, 160, 11–20. Available at: <http://linkinghub.elsevier.com/retrieve/pii/S0093934X15300845> (Accessed 14 October, 2017).

Feld, J. E., & Sommers, M. S. (2009). Lipreading, processing speed, and working memory in younger and older adults. *J. Speech Lang. Hear. Res.*, 52, 1555–1565 Available at: <http://jslhr.pubs.asha.org/article.aspx?doi=10.1044/1092-43882009/08-0137)> (Accessed 1 November, 2018).

Ferjan Ramirez, N., Leonard, M. K., Davenport, T. S., Torres, C., Halgren, E., & Mayberry, R. I. (2016). Neural language processing in adolescent first-language learners: Longitudinal case studies in American Sign Language. *Cereb. Cortex*, 26(3), 1015–1026. doi: doi: https://doi.org/10.1093/cercor/bhu273

Ferjan Ramirez, N., Leonard, M. K., Torres, C., Hatrak, M., Halgren, E., & Mayberry, R. I. (2014). Neural language processing in adolescent first-language learners. *Cereb. Cortex*, 24, 2772–2783 Available at: <http://www.ncbi.nlm.nih.gov/pubmed/23696277> (Accessed 31 October, 2018).

Finney, E. M., Fine, I., Dobkins, K. R. (2001). Visual stimuli activate auditory cortex in the deaf. *Nat. Neurosci*, 4, 1171–1173 Available at: <http://www.ncbi.nlm.nih.gov/pubmed/11704763>

Gathercole, S. E., & Baddeley, A. D. (1993). *Working memory and language.* Hove: Psychology Press.

Glick, H., & Sharma, A. (2017). Cross-modal plasticity in developmental and age-related hearing loss: Clinical implications. *Hear. Res.*, 343, 191–201. Available at: <http://www.ncbi.nlm.nih.gov/pubmed/27613397> (Accessed November, 2018).

Gutierrez-Sigut, E., Daws, R., Payne, H., Blott, J., Marshall, C., & MacSweeney, M. (2015). Language lateralization of hearing native signers: A functional transcranial Doppler sonography (fTCD) study of speech and sign production. *Brain Lang.*, 151, 23–34 Available at: <http://linkinghub.elsevier.com/retrieve/pii/S0093934X15300870> (Accessed 14 October, 2017).

Gutierrez-Sigut, E., Payne, H., & MacSweeney, M. (2016). Examining the contribution of motor movement and language dominance to increased left lateralization during sign generation in native signers. *Brain Lang.*, 159, 109–117 Available at: <http://linkinghub.elsevier.com/retrieve/pii/S0093934X16300402> (Accessed 14 October, 2017).

Hensch, T. K. (2004). Critical period regulation. *Annu. Rev. Neurosci.*, 27, 549–579. Available at: <http://www.ncbi.nlm.nih.gov/pubmed/15217343> (Accessed 26 May, 2014).

Hickok, G., Bellugi, U., & Klima, E. S. (1996). The neurobiology of sign language and its implications for the neural basis of language. *Nature*, 381, 699–702. Available at: <http://www.ncbi.nlm.nih.gov/pubmed/8649515>

Hickok, G., & Poeppel, D. (2007). The cortical organization of speech processing. *Nat. Rev. Neurosci.*, 8, 393–402 Available at: <http://www.nature.com/nrn/journal/v8/n5/abs/nrn2113.html> (Accessed 20 June, 2014).

Holland, S. K., Vannest, J., Mecoli, M., Jacola, L. M., Tillema, J.-M., Karunanayaka, P. R., Schmithorst, V. J., Yuan, W., Plante, E., & Byars, A. W. (2007). Functional MRI of language lateralization during development in children. *Int. J. Audiol.*, 46, 533–551. Available at: <http://www.ncbi.nlm.nih.gov/pubmed/17828669> (Accessed 1 November, 2018).

Holmer, E., Heimann, M., & Rudner, M. (2016). Imitation, sign language skill and the developmental ease of language understanding (D-ELU) model. *Front. Psychol.*, 7. Available at: <http://journal.frontiersin.org/Article/10.3389/fpsyg.2016.00107/abstract> (Accessed 3 October, 2017).

Hornsby, B. W. Y. (2013). The effects of hearing aid use on listening effort and mental fatigue associated with sustained speech processing demands. *Ear Hear.*, 34, 523–534 Available at: <http://content.wkhealth.com/linkback/openurl?sid=WKPTLP:landingpage&an=00003446-201309000-00001> (Accessed 31 October, 2018).

Karns, C. M., Dow, M. W., & Neville, H. J. (2012. Altered cross-modal processing in the primary auditory cortex of congenitally deaf adults: A visual-somatosensory fMRI study with a double-flash illusion. *J. Neurosci.*, 32, 9626–9638.

Kral, A. (2013). Auditory critical periods: A review from system's perspective. *Neuroscience*, 247, 117–133. Available at: <https://www.sciencedirect.com/science/article/pii/S0306452213004338> (Accessed 26 June, 2018).

Kyle, F. E., Campbell, R., Mohammed, T., Coleman, M., & Macsweeney, M. (2013). Speechreading development in deaf and hearing children: Introducing the test of child speechreading. *J. Speech Lang. Hear. Res.*, 5, 16–426. Available at: <http://jslhr.pubs.asha.org/article.aspx?doi=10.1044/1092-4388(2012/12-0039)>(Accessed 14 October, 2017).

Lenneberg, E. H. (1967). *Biological foundations of language*. New York, NY: John Wiley and Sons.

Leonard, M. K., Ferjan-Ramirez, N., Torres, C., Travis, K. E., Hatrak, M., Mayberry, R., & Halgren, E. (2012). Signed words in the congenitally deaf evoke typical late lexicosemantic responses with no early visual responses in left superior temporal cortex. *J. Neurosci.*, 32, 9700–9705.

Lomber, S. G., Meredith, M. A. , & Kral, A. (2010). Cross-modal plasticity in specific auditory cortices underlies visual compensations in the deaf. *Nat. Neurosci.*, 13, 1421–1427. Available at: <http://www.ncbi.nlm.nih.gov/pubmed/2093564>

Ludman, C., Summerfield, A. Q., Hall, D., Elliott, M., Fostevr, J., Hykin, J., Bowtell, R., & Morris, P. (2000). Lip-reading ability and patterns of cortical activation studied using fMRI. *Br. J. Audiol.*, 34, 225–230.

Lyness, C. R., Woll, B., Campbell, R., & Cardin, V. (2013). How does visual language affect cross-modal plasticity and cochlear implant success? *Neurosci. Biobehav. Rev.*, 37, 2621–2630.

MacSweeney, M., Campbell, R., Woll, B., Giampietro, V., David, A. S., McGuire, P. K., Calvert, G. A, & Brammer, M. J. (2004). Dissociating linguistic and nonlinguistic gestural communication in the brain. *Neuroimage*, 22, 1605–1618. Available at: <http://www.ncbi.nlm.nih.gov/pubmed/15275917> (Accessed 27 May, 2014).

MacSweeney, M., Capek, C. M., Campbell, R., & Woll, B. (2008a). The signing brain: The neurobiology of sign language. *Trends Cog. Sci.*, 12, 432–440. Available at: <http://www.ncbi.nlm.nih.gov/pubmed/18805728>

MacSweeney, M., Waters, D., Brammer, M. J., Woll, B., & Goswami, U. (2008b). Phonological processing in deaf signers and the impact of age of first language acquisition. *Neuroimage*, 40, 1369–1379.

MacSweeney, M., Woll, B., Campbell, R., Calvert, G. A., McGuire, P. K., David, A. S., Simmons, A., & Brammer, M. J. (2002a). Neural correlates of British sign language comprehension: Spatial processing demands of topographic language. *J. Cogn. Neurosci.*, 14, 1064–1075 Available at: <http://www.ncbi.nlm.nih.gov/pubmed/12419129> (Accessed 14 October, 2017).

MacSweeney, M., Woll, B., Campbell, R., McGuire, P. K., David, A. S., Williams, S. C. R., Suckling, J., Calvert, G. A., Brammer, M. J. (2002b). Neural systems underlying British Sign Language and audio-visual English processing in native users. *Brain*, 125, 1583–1593 Available at: <http://www.ncbi.nlm.nih.gov/pubmed/12077007>

Marshall, C., Jones, A., Denmark, T., Mason, K., Atkinson, J., Botting, N., & Morgan, G. (2015). Deaf children's non-verbal working memory is impacted by their language experience. *Front. Psychol.*, 6, 527. Available at: <http://www.pubmedcentral.nih.gov/articlerender.fcgi?artid=4419661&tool=pmcentrez&rendertype=abstract> (Accessed 8 October, 2015).

Marshall, J., Atkinson, J., Woll, B., & Thacker, A. (2005). Aphasia in a bilingual user of British signlanguage and english: Effects of cross-linguistic cues. *Cogn. Neuropsychol.*, 22, 719–736 Available at: <http://www.tandfonline.com/doi/abs/10.1080/02643290442000266> (Accessed 14 October, 2017).

Mayberry, R. I., Chen, J.-K., Witcher, P., & Klein, D. (2011). Age of acquisition effects on the functional organization of language in the adult brain. *Brain Lang.*, 119, 16–29 Available at: <http://www.ncbi.nlm.nih.gov/pubmed/21705060> (Accessed 28 May, 2014).

Mayberry, R. I., Lock, E., & Kazmi, H. (2002). Linguistic ability and early language exposure. *Nature*, 417, 38 Available at: <http://www.ncbi.nlm.nih.gov/pubmed/11986658>

McCullough, S., Saygin, A. P., Korpics, F., & Emmorey, K. (2012). Motion-sensitive cortex and motion semantics in American Sign Language. *Neuroimage*, 63, 111–118. Available at: <http://linkinghub.elsevier.com/retrieve/pii/S105381191200643X> (Accessed 14 October, 2017).

Mayberry R. I., Lock E. (2003 Dec). Age constraints on first versus second language acquisition: evidence for linguistic plasticity and epigenesis. *Brain Lang* 87(3), 369–84.

Merabet, L. B., & Pascual-Leone, A. (2010). Neural reorganization following sensory loss: The opportunity of change. *Nat. Rev. Neurosci.*, 11, 44–52. Available at: <http://www.ncbi.nlm.nih.gov/pubmed/19935836>

Mercure, E., Kushnerenko, E., Goldberg L., Bowden-Howl, H., Coulson, K., Johnson, M. H., & MacSweeney, M. (2018). Language experience influences audiovisual speech integration in unimodal and bimodal bilingual infants. *Dev. Sci*, e12701 Available at: <http://doi.wiley.com/10.1111/desc.12701> (Accessed 31 October, 2018).

Mohammed, T., Campbell, R., Macsweeney, M., Barry, F., & Coleman, M. (2006). Speechreading and its association with reading among deaf, hearing and dyslexic individuals. In *Clinical linguistics and phonetics* (pp. 621–630). Available at: <http://www.ncbi.nlm.nih.gov/pubmed/17056494> (Accessed 14 October, 2017).

Neville, H. J., & Bavelier, D. (1998). Neural organization and plasticity of language. *Curr. Opin. Neurobiol.*, 8, 254–258. Available at: <http://www.ncbi.nlm.nih.gov/pubmed/9635210> (Accessed 1 November, 2018).

Newman, A. J., Supalla, T., Fernandez, N., Newport, E. L., & Bavelier, D. (2015). Neural systems supporting linguistic structure, linguistic experience, and symbolic communication in sign language and gesture. *Proc. Natl. Acad. Sci.*, 112, 11684–11689. Available at: <http://www.ncbi.nlm.nih.gov/pubmed/26283352> (Accessed 14 October, 2017).

Nishimura, H., Hashikawa, K., Doi, K., Iwaki, T., Watanabe, Y., Kusuoka, H., Nishimura, T., & Kubo, T. (1999). Sign language "heard" in the auditory cortex *Nature*, 397, 116 Available at: <http://www.ncbi.nlm.nih.gov/pubmed/9923672>

Pa, J., Wilson, S. M., Pickell, H., Bellugi, U., & Hickok, G. (2009). Neural organization of linguistic short-term memory is sensory modality-dependent: Evidence from signed and spoken language. *Journal of Cognitive Neuroscience*, 20(12), 2198–2210.

Pierce, L. J., Genesee, F., Delcenserie, A., & Morgan, G. (2017). Variations in phonological working memory: Linking early language experiences and language learning outcomes. *Appl. Psycholinguist.*, 38, 1265–1300 Available at: <https://www.cambridge.org/core/product/identifier/S0142716417000236/type/journal_article> (Accessed 16 March, 2018).

Rauschecker, J. P., & Scott, S. K. (2009). Maps and streams in the auditory cortex: Nonhuman primates illuminate human speech processing. *Nat. Neurosci.*, 12, 718–724 Available at: <http://www.ncbi.nlm.nih.gov/pubmed/19471271>

Röder, B., Stock, O., Bien, S., Neville, H., & Rösler, F. (2002). Speech processing activates visual cortex in congenitally blind humans. *Eur. J. Neurosci.*, 16, 930–936. Available at: <http://www.ncbi.nlm.nih.gov/pubmed/12372029> (Accessed 2 August, 2016).

Rönnberg, J., Holmer, E., & Rudner, M. (2019). Cognitive hearing science and ease of language understanding. *International Journal of Audiology.* Doi https://doi.org/10.1080/14992027.2018.1551631 [Epub ahead of print].

Rönnberg, J., Lunner, T., Zekveld, A., Sörqvist, P., Danielsson, H., Lyxell, B., Dahlström, Ö., Signoret, C., Stenfelt, S., Pichora-Fuller, M. K., & Rudner, M. (2013). The Ease of Language Understanding (ELU) model: Theoretical, empirical, and clinical advances. *Front. Syst. Neurosci.*, 7. Available at: <http://journal.frontiersin.org/article/10.3389/fnsys.2013.00031/abstract> (Accessed 3 October, 2017).

Rönnberg, J., Rudner, M., & Ingvar, M. (2004). Neural correlates of working memory for sign language. *Brain Res. Cogn. Brain Res.*, 20, 165–182 Available at: <http://www.ncbi.nlm.nih.gov/pubmed/15183389> (Accessed 28 May, 2014).

Rudner, M. (2015). Working memory for meaningless manual gestures. *Can. J. Exp. Psychol. Can. Psychol. Expérimentale*, 69, 72–79. Available at: <http://doi.apa.org/getdoi.cfm?doi=10.1037/cep0000033> (Accessed 3 October, 2017).

Rudner, M. (2018). Working memory for linguistic and non-linguistic manual gestures: Evidence, theory, and application. *Front. Psychol.*, 9, 679.

Rudner, M., Foo, C., Rönnberg, J., & Lunner, T. (2009). Cognition and aided speech recognition in noise: Specific role for cognitive factors following nine-week experience with adjusted compression settings in hearing aids. *Scan. J. Psychol.*, 50, 405–418.

Rudner, M., Fransson, P., Ingvar, M., Nyberg, L., & Rönnberg, J. (2007.) Neural representation of binding lexical signs and words in the episodic buffer of working memory. *Neuropsychologia*, 45, 2258–2276. Available at: <http://www.ncbi.nlm.nih.gov/pubmed/17403529> (Accessed 16 June, 2014).

Rudner, M., Karlsson, T., Gunnarsson, J., & Rönnberg, J. (2013). Levels of processing and language modality specificity in working memory. *Neuropsychologia*, 51, 656–666 Available at: <http://www.ncbi.nlm.nih.gov/pubmed/23287569> (Accessed 24 May, 2014).

Rudner, M., Orfanidou, E., Cardin, V., Capek, C. M., Woll, B., & Rönnberg, J. (2016). Preexisting semantic representation improves working memory performance in the visuospatial domain. *Mem. Cognit.*, 44, 608–620. Available at: <http://link.springer.com/10.3758/s13421-016-0585-z> (Accessed 3 October, 2017).

Rudner, M., & Rönnberg, J. (2019). Working memory for signs and gestures. In M. Marschark & P. E. Spencer, Oxford handbook of deaf studies in language. Oxford: Oxford University Press.

Rudner, M., & Rönnberg, J. (2008). The role of the episodic buffer in working memory for language processing. *Cogn. Process.*, 9, 19–28. Available at: <http://www.ncbi.nlm.nih.gov/pubmed/17917753> (Accessed 16 June, 2014).

Signoret, C., Johnsrude, I., Classon, E., & Rudner, M. (2018). Combined effects of form- and meaning-based predictability on perceived clarity of speech. *J. Exp. Psychol. Hum. Percept. Perform.*, 44, 277–285. Available at: <http://doi.apa.org/getdoi.cfm?doi=10.1037/xhp0000442> (Accessed 3 October, 2017).

Söderfeldt, B., Ingvar, M., Rönnberg, J., Eriksson, L., Serrander, M., & Stone-Elander, S. (1997). Signed and spoken language perception studied by positron emission tomography. *Neurology*, 49, 82–87. Available at: <http://www.ncbi.nlm.nih.gov/pubmed/9222174>

Sorqvist, P., & Rönnberg, J. (2012). Episodic long-term memory of spoken discourse masked by speech: What is the role for working memory capacity? *J. Speech Lang. Hear. Res.*, 55, 210–218.

Sutton-Spence, R., & Woll, B. (1999). *The linguistics of British Sign Language: An introduction*. Cambridge: Cambridge University Press.

Tamati, T. N., Gilbert, J. L., & Pisoni, D. B. (2013). Some factors underlying individual differences in speech recognition on PRESTO: A first report. *J. Am. Acad. Audiol.*, 24, 616–634 Available at: <http://openurl.ingenta.com/content/xref?genre=article&issn=1050-0545&volume=24&issue=7&spage=616> (Accessed 14 October, 2017).

Twomey, T., Waters, D., Price, C. J., Evans, S., & MacSweeney, M. (2017). How auditory experience differentially influences the function of left and right superior temporal cortices. *J. Neurosci.*, 37, 9564–9573 Available at: <http://www.jneurosci.org/lookup/doi/10.1523/JNEUROSCI.0846-17.2017> (Accessed 14 October, 2017).

Venezia, J. H., Vaden, K. I., Rong, F., Maddox, D., Saberi, K., & Hickok, G. (2017). Auditory, visual and audiovisual speech processing streams in superior temporal sulcus. *Front. Hum. Neurosci.*, 11. Available at: <http://journal.frontiersin.org/article/10.3389/fnhum.2017.00174/full> (Accessed 4 October, 2017).

Wilson, M. (2001). The case for sensorimotor coding in working memory. *Psychon. Bull. Rev.*, 8, 44–57. Available at: <http://www.ncbi.nlm.nih.gov/pubmed/11340866> (Accessed 4 October, 2017).

Wilson, M., & Emmorey, K. (1997). A visuospatial "phonological loop" in working memory: Evidence from American Sign Language. *Mem. Cognit.*, 25, 313–320. Available at: <http://www.ncbi.nlm.nih.gov/pubmed/9184483> (Accessed 3 October, 2017).

Zosh, J. M., & Feigenson, L. (2015). Array heterogeneity prevents catastrophic forgetting in infants. *Cognition*, 136, 365–380 Available at: <https://linkinghub.elsevier.com/retrieve/pii/S0010027714002686> (Accessed 31 October, 2018).

CHAPTER 10

Educating bilingual and multilingual deaf children in the 21st century

Gladys Tang, Robert Adam and Karen Simpson OBE

This chapter offers an overview of sign bilingual education and some of the complex issues and challenges that impacted the evolution of sign bilingual practices in Europe, Australia and Asia. One such challenge is the promotion of inclusive education in recent years, which triggers a new thinking of partnering sign bilingualism with co-enrolment education for deaf and hearing children. The chapter ends with a summary of factors surrounding the future development of sign bilingual education, from the perspective of empirical research and pedagogy.

1. Introduction

The advent of research into the linguistics of sign languages from the 1960s and the concern for persistently low linguistic and academic outcomes of deaf students who were educated orally helped to raise the profile of sign languages in educational settings as naturally evolving languages in the 1980s (Plaza-Pust, 2012). Interest in sign bilingual education for deaf children subsequently developed in many parts of the world – initially in Europe and North America, and later in Australia and Asia.

The primary aim of sign bilingual education, especially when it was first introduced in the 1980s, was to promote the acquisition of sign language as a first or dominant language for deaf children, followed by the development of a spoken language once a strong sign language foundation was established. Additionally, emphasis was on developing deaf children's reading and writing skills in the ambient spoken language of society, while it was well understood that speech development was often dependent on individual potentials and the effectiveness of assistive hearing technology. Due to technological advances and changes in our societies, sign bilingual programmes can become more flexible and responsive to the individual linguistic repertoires and learning needs of deaf children and young people (Swanwick, 2017).

https://doi.org/10.1075/tilar.25.10tan

Philosophically, bilingual education in the 21st century strives towards the humanitarian and democratic goals of social inclusion and diversity. In the deaf education context, it is an approach to education that recognizes the unique and distinctive features of the languages and cultures of deaf people, validates the linguistic and cultural choices of deaf people, and celebrates this diversity (Ainscow, 2005). Although most deaf children do not enter the school system until 4 to 5 years of age in many parts of the world, this mode of education aspires to provide full access to a language for learning and development as early as possible. As such, delay in language development is never acceptable for deaf children, and early exposure to sign language is perceived to be their linguistic human right.[1] Moreover, deaf children should be granted access to a curriculum in whichever language that is most accessible to them, in an environment that values deafness, sign language and deaf culture.

This chapter has several aims. Firstly, we offer an overview of sign bilingual education in countries that we are familiar with, explore some of the complex issues and challenges raised over the last few decades, and identify how these have impacted the evolution of sign bilingual practices. Secondly, we present some new developments in sign bilingual education, demonstrating how the concept of sign bilingualism may be modified and implemented effectively, especially in 'inclusive' or co-enrollment programmes for deaf and hearing children in mainstream settings. Thirdly, we consider the changing linguistic repertoires of deaf children in the world of technology nowadays, surrounded by increasingly multi-lingual and multi-cultural societies. Fourthly, we provide a summary of factors surrounding the future development of sign bilingual education, from the perspective of empirical research and pedagogy. We argue that fundamental research is still sorely needed, focusing not only on the linguistic properties of sign language and how they are acquired and processed, but also on the optimum conditions for developing effective sign bilingual practices that purposefully attempt to bring natural sign language in to different educational contexts. In addition, this chapter explores ways in which the new knowledge generated from both sign linguistics and deaf education research can be disseminated to school communities to strengthen and improve teaching practices in deaf education.

2. The evolution of sign bilingual education in three continents

In this section, we will focus on the evolution of sign bilingual education programmes implemented in the UK, Australia and Asia.

---

1. <https://wfdeaf.org/news/wfd-position-paper-language-rights-deaf-children/>

2.1 UK

The landscape for schools for deaf children and deaf education in the UK has changed dramatically over the last 30 years. In 1983, an organization – The Language of Sign as an Educational Resource (LASER) – was established to explore the possibilities of using sign language in educational settings. LASER challenged the misconception that being sign bilingual was a disadvantage, based on the observation that deaf children of deaf parents with early exposure to sign language were educationally more successful than those deaf children with hearing parents. Alongside this, there was a growing dissatisfaction with the dominant oralist approach, in particular the poor achievement of deaf learners as evidenced by Conrad's study of deaf school leavers in the 1970's (Conrad, 1979). The LASER project was summarized in Pickersgill and Gregory (1998) in which the philosophy, policy and practice of 'sign bilingualism' were laid out with practical examples. During that time, two schools for deaf children and one service started to embrace such a concept: the Royal School for the Deaf, Derby and Longwill School in Birmingham, and the deaf and hearing impaired (DAHISS) service in Leeds Local Authority. Later on in the 1990s, several other schools for deaf children, and some resource bases and services followed suit by adopting a sign bilingual approach in the classroom. Teachers of the Deaf (ToDs) working in these schools and services felt empowered by having a language – British Sign Language (BSL) – that they could use to deliver the curriculum, which the children could access and understand easily. Also, as the sign bilingual approach recognized the importance of deaf culture and identity, it encouraged the involvement of deaf as well as hearing people in the education of deaf children. As a result, deaf people were increasingly employed in these schools and served as linguistic and cultural role models as well as educators. Consequently over time ToDs observed significant developments in deaf children's self-esteem and sense of deaf identity in such settings. Such schools further developed their teaching strategies and created teaching resources to enable deaf children to achieve their full potential. The Sign Bilingual Consortium (SBC) of deaf schools and services was established in 1998 to share this good practice through networking and training. As recognition of BSL and the role it played in deaf education steadily grew, more vocational BSL courses were introduced by the Council for the Advancement of Communication with Deaf People (now Signature[2]), which enabled hearing ToDs and support staff to obtain qualifications in BSL, potentially to interpreter level. Some of these mandatory ToD courses offered a specific focus on sign bilingual issues, which was of particular importance to ToDs teaching in these sign bilingual schools and

---

2. <www.signature.org.uk>

services. New tools were developed to assess deaf children's expressive and receptive BSL skills (see Herman et al, this volume). As a result, there was an increasing number of deaf ToDs and well-qualified deaf professionals working in deaf education. Eventually BSL was recognised as an official language by the Department of Work and Pensions of the British Government in March 2003.

However, over the thirty years in which sign bilingual education has developed, the context both within education and for deaf people has changed dramatically. Within education, an emphasis on inclusive practice grew and increasingly more deaf children began to attend their local mainstream schools and resource bases (see CRIDE, 2011 & 2017 reports below). This situation was aggravated by the implementation of the revised *Special Educational Needs and Disability Code of Practice (SEND, 2015)*, where local authorities have striven to reduce the number of out-of-borough (out of state or region) placements they fund for children with SEND in England. As such, it has become more preferable for deaf children to be educated in a mainstream school within their council borough as opposed to being sent to a school for deaf children or a resource base in another borough. This has led to a reduction in requests for placements of sign bilingual deaf children in many deaf schools. When requests are actually made, they are for those deaf children with a much more complex range of learning needs that cannot be met in-borough. This trend is evidenced in the Consortium for Research into Deaf Education (CRIDE, 2011 and 2017)[3] survey reports. In the 2011 CRIDE report for England, 73% of school-aged deaf children were in mainstream settings with no specialist provision, 8% were in mainstream schools with resource provision, 6% attended special schools for deaf children or independent schools, and 12% attended other special schools. In the 2017 CRIDE UK-wide report, the number of school-aged deaf children attending mainstream schools with no specialist provision had increased to 78%, those attending mainstream schools with resource provisions had decreased to 6%, the number attending special schools for deaf children had also decreased to 3%, and the number attending special schools (not specifically for deaf children) remained static.

Early identification of deafness through the Newborn Hearing Screening Programme (NHSP) was introduced across England since 2002 and came into full force in March 2006. It coupled with advancement in digital technology, opening up visual and text-based communication among deaf and hearing people, including access to the internet, email, social media, SMS/mobile phones, tablets, BSL TV channels and subtitling on television (Power, Power, & Horstmanshof, 2007). Digital hearing aids and FM systems, and especially cochlear implantation (CI) as young as 12 months, have enabled many severe to profoundly deaf children to

---

3. <http://www.ndcs.org.uk/professional_support/national_data/cride.html>

develop functional hearing and spoken language to some extent. CIs were introduced in the UK at about the same time as sign bilingual education was in the early
1990s. As such, ToDs in sign bilingual deaf schools now witness young implanted
deaf children using BSL to support them to acquire fluent spoken English until
they reach a point when they are truly bilingual and can move flexibly between
the two languages. In the UK, 28% of school-aged deaf children (0–19) use sign
language 'in some form' either as their sole language (7%) or alongside another
language (21%). Furthermore, in this context, 13% of deaf learners use spoken
languages at home other than English (CRIDE, 2017). Deaf young people who
have implants and also sign tend to feel more at ease with language choice dependent on needs of the situation rather than particular language practices (Wheeler
et al., 2007). As a result, where the society is becoming increasingly diverse and
multi-lingual, it is now possible to observe more frequent multimodal use of
languages by deaf children, especially in sign bilingual deaf schools. This has led
to the development of a new theoretical model of deaf bimodal bilingualism that
recognizes the plural and diverse communicative resources of deaf children and
young people (Swanwick, 2017). Consequently, several deaf schools in the UK
have adopted the term 'bi- or multilingualism' to describe their educational and
communication philosophy and practice as they believe this reflects the diverse
language repertoires of their learners.

Since 2011, teaching practitioners in the UK have been able to access de-
mographic data on provision and educational support for deaf children through
the CRIDE annual survey reports. Currently, CRIDE is working in collaboration
with National Sensory Impairment Partnership (NatSIP), UCL, City University
London, and the University of London by undertaking a 7-year longitudinal
study of individual pupils with data collection funded by the Ovingdean Hall
Foundation for the first 3 years. The purpose of the longitudinal study is to investigate the relationships between pupil, provision, participation variables and
outcomes with the overall aim of improving provision and outcomes for deaf
children and young people.

2.2   Australia

In Australia, adopting sign language in educating deaf children has a long history
and was synonymous with early deaf education since Thomas Pattison opened the
first school for deaf children in Sydney in 1860 and Frederick John Rose established
the school for deaf children in Melbourne in the same year (Burchett, 1964). BSL,
which later evolved into what is now known as Australian Sign Language (Auslan),
was used as a language of instruction in both schools. Other signing schools for
deaf children were established in Brisbane in 1893 (Carty, 2004). Johnston and

Schembri (2007) describe a succession of teachers, missionaries and others who arrived in Australia from Britain, all of whom used BSL. However, in the 1870s, children studying in the Melbourne School for the deaf began to be separated between oral and signing, and lip reading and speech training were introduced. Since the 1890s, the 'combined method' (i.e. sign and speech) has been used at school, and is still used at present. A similar evolution from pure signing to the 'combined method' occurred in the school for the deaf in Sydney, in the midst of the increasingly common practice of mainstreaming deaf students or opening of oral schools for the deaf in various cities (Burchett, op.cit.). Towards the 1970s, there were more deaf children being placed in mainstream settings and so the Visiting Teacher Service was established in Melbourne to support the children in these schools. Later in this period, there was also a perceived need to standardize the sign language used by the deaf community in Australia and so an 'Aid to communication with the Deaf' was published in 1972, followed by two editions of the Dictionary of Australasian signs published in 1982 and 1989. This was the precursor of the publication of the first Auslan dictionary in 1989, during a time when the Deaf community became more aware of its linguistic status. In 1984, sign language interpreters were invited into the mainstream classroom. The National Languages Policy in 1989 saw the acknowledgement of Auslan as a community language. It was also during that time that the first sign bilingual education programme, which used both Auslan and English, was established officially by the Royal Institute for Deaf and Blind Children in New South Wales at the Roberta Reid Centre in 1992, an early childhood centre, followed by the establishment of the Thomas Pattison School in 1993. In Victoria, the Victorian School for Deaf Children (now the Victorian College for the Deaf) followed suit and adopted a sign bilingual philosophy.

In 2001 a survey report on sign bilingual education was issued by the Department of Education of the South Australian government, who analyzed the sign bilingual practices of nine model schools, according to the principles of assimilation, pluralism, synthesis, separation, and segregation. They identified that there was a variety of sign bilingual practices in both schools for the deaf and mainstream schools. As well as conventional sign bilingual practices they observed 'reversed integration with deaf schools', such as Brighton Primary School in Adelaide, in which a critical mass of hearing children, children with hearing loss, and deaf students are placed in classes together and taught by ToDs using English and Auslan. According to the survey report, this model of 'reversed integration' follows the philosophy and practices of 'co-enrollment' in deaf education (Kirchner, 1994). In this model, to support students with their learning, it is the state government that provides funding for a Deaf Instructor to support the sign language development of deaf students and for sign interpretation by an interpreter or a ToD. In 2017, the Australian Curriculum, Assessment and Reporting Authority introduced an AUSLAN curriculum for all school stages (i.e., kindergarten through K12) based on two pathways: (a) First Language Learner for deaf children and hearing children of deaf parents, and (b) Second Language Learner for children who did not learn AUSLAN from their parents).[4] This policy at least strengthens the concepts of sign bilingualism for school age students deaf children.

2.3   Asia

The spread of sign bilingual education across Asia in the 1980s and 1990s was not as systematic or extensive compared to Europe or the US. This was primarily due to a lack of sign linguistics and sign language acquisition research during that period to validate and encourage its development. As a result, schools for deaf children in Japan, Korea, Taiwan, Hong Kong, and China, have maintained either an oralist or Total Communication philosophy, due to the impact of medical and technological advancement as well as newborn hearing screening. In many of these schools where signing is accepted, the ToDs prioritize manually coded spoken languages over the natural sign languages of the Deaf communities in educating deaf children (Jhang, 2015; Yang, 2008). As a consequence, the two modes of communication co-exist in the deaf school context. In China, for instance, the education policy supports oral education for deaf children, thus it is quite common to find very young pre-school deaf children receiving an oral education initially, and manually-coded signed language is gradually introduced into the classroom during primary education.

In Cambodia, deaf education from Grade 1 to Grade 12 is arranged by a non-government organization called Krousar Thmey. While signing is accepted at school, ToDs use either signs taken from American Sign Language or an artificial signing system called 'Khmer Sign Language' to teach from textbooks written in Khmer. This mixed use of signing varieties differs from the local indigenous Cambodian Sign Language which is currently under documentation.

However, even in the absence of sign linguistics research, some form of sign bilingual education exists in some developing countries, especially in those where universal screening and early intervention with advanced hearing assistive technology are not so well established. In Sri Lanka, for instance, schools for the deaf play an important role in supporting deaf children's elementary education (Hettiarachchi et al., in press). This suggests that sign language support is incorporated into the education system for the deaf in Sri Lanka; however, the involvement of deaf teachers remains low. Also, in spite of the efforts of the government,

---

4. <https://www.australiancurriculum.edu.au/f-10-curriculum/languages/auslan/>

there are still deaf individuals in Sri Lanka who have never received any formal education and who use gestures or home signs to communicate.

Similarly to western countries, the existence of sign linguists locally in Asia has encouraged the establishment of sign bilingual programmes. In Vietnam, the high school programme – the Dong Nai Deaf Education Project (2000 to 2012) – reported in Woodward and Nguyen (2012) recognizes the use of Ho Chi Ming City Sign Language (HCMCSL) as the main language of instruction as adult deaf students come from various parts of the country use different signing varieties. Although the majority of teachers are hearing in this programme, they learn HCMCSL in order to teach curriculum subjects to their deaf students. In Japan, linguistic research on Japanese Sign Language has led to the establishment of Meisei Gakuen School for the Deaf in 2008. It is a private school from kindergarten to junior secondary 4 and adopts a sign bilingual approach. In China, there were individual attempts to establish sign bilingual education between 1996 and 2014 through the SignAm Project, due to concerns over the effectiveness of Signed Chinese and Chinese Pinyin in deaf education. From the school for deaf children in Nanjing, the approach spread to Suzhou, Changzhou, Zhengjiang, Yanzhou, and subsequently four schools for the deaf in Sichuan and Guizhou Provinces (Wu et al., 2005). Another attempt was launched by the UNICEF's Bilingual-Bicultural Programme (2001–2008) which also focused primarily on developing sign bilingual provision for pre-school deaf children within a deaf school context. It founded bases in Tianjin and Chengdu, plus a speech/language rehabilitation centre in Foshan of Guangdong Province (Wu, 2008). Like the SignAm project, deaf teachers were recruited to support the sign language acquisition of deaf children because most parents were hearing, and sign language was viewed as the dominant or preferred language. There were also attempts to integrate one or two deaf children into a mainstream classroom at the end of the project, where these children were accompanied by a Deaf teacher working as a teaching aid.

Turning to Hong Kong, sign bilingual education for deaf children has never been formulated as a government policy. Formal deaf education began in 1935 with the establishment of the Hong Kong School for the Deaf which adopted a strict oralist approach. During the post WWII period, seven more schools for deaf children were established among which two promoted sign bilingual education. These two schools were supervised by Deaf teachers who came from Nanjing and Shanghai and who brought with them the signing varieties from those cities. According to Sze et al. (2013), these varieties laid the foundation for the development of Hong Kong Sign Language (HKSL). Also during the late 1960s, the Social Welfare Department of the government set up six 'clubs for deaf children' and promoted using the signing varieties from these two deaf schools to support the early development of pre-school deaf children. When the responsibility of educating deaf children was shifted from the Social Welfare Department to the Education Department in the 1970s, sign bilingual education began to wane and oralist education took its place, or Total Communication in one deaf school. Between 2003 and 2006, following research on the linguistics of HKSL, a sign bilingual programme was trialled in the deaf school that only accepted Total Communication. Its aim was to boost the Chinese literacy skills of deaf children through the support of Deaf teachers who used HKSL during the Chinese lessons (Tang, Chan, & Chan, 2006). Although improvement in Chinese literacy was observed, the school decided to revert back to a Total Communication philosophy when the project expired in 2006. In summary, the development of sign bilingual education in Asia was not as systematic as what had happened in the UK or Australia. The main impetus for change probably came from the introduction of the UN Convention on the Rights of Persons with Disabilities (CRPD) (United Nations, 2006), which affirms the linguistic status of sign language and the rights of deaf children to receive education in sign language. The CRPD has also led to the official recognition in legislation of sign languages in some countries like Thailand and Korea. For Hong Kong there was an unsuccessful attempt in 2017 to recognize HKSL in legislation as one of the official languages on a par with Cantonese, English and written Chinese.

3. Sign bilingual education in practice – Issues and challenges

As with any new innovation, the implementation of sign bilingual education has not been without its critics or challenges. Knoors and Marschark (2012) argue that the term 'sign bilingual education' sometimes invokes different interpretations and even practices, especially regarding the quality of the language of instruction. In order to provide a fluent sign language as a language of instruction, a high level of signing proficiency is expected of practitioners. However, the great majority of ToDs are hearing and adult learners of sign language, and have diverse sign language skills and ideologies about different signing varieties. In some western countries, this issue has been addressed by schools for the deaf ensuring that there are both native sign language practitioners and hearing practitioners teaching collaboratively in classes, and by establishing sign language teaching centres, offering accredited courses for children, practitioners and parents.

The advancement in assistive hearing technology such as digital hearing aids and cochlear implantation has resulted in documented improvement in hearing levels for many deaf children. This has prompted debate over the necessity for and the role of sign language in deaf education, especially how it enhances or impedes spoken language development. A controversial paper by Geers et al.'s (2017) claims that implanted deaf children with long-term exposure to sign language produced less intelligible speech, had lower speech perception and a slower development of spoken language when compared with non-signing children. Nevertheless, there have already been studies emphasizing early exposure to sign language by deaf children, even before potential cochlear implantation, to guard against missing the critical period of language acquisition (Humphries et al., 2014; Napoli et al., 2015).

Other areas of ongoing debate have been about the pedagogical effectiveness of natural sign language and manually coded spoken language in sign bilingual education. Related to this is the 'lack of transfer' view between sign language and spoken language in supporting deaf children's literacy development, on grounds that the diverse phonological knowledge between sign language and spoken language makes transfer impracticable if not impossible (Mayer & Leigh, 2010). This argument however, is based solely on a phonological model of the reading process and does not take into account other routes or components contributing to literacy development such as vocabulary knowledge, grammatical knowledge and inferential skills (Hermans et al., 2010; Tang et al., 2014).

As observed earlier in this chapter, a major factor influencing the development of sign bilingual education is the widespread change of educational philosophy from segregation to integration or 'inclusion' in deaf education. This philosophy has resulted in a significant shift of educational context where many deaf children are being placed in mainstream education instead of schools for the deaf, where access to sign language, Deaf peers, and Deaf teachers are largely unprovided for. The rise of 'inclusive' education has led to a rapid reduction in the number of schools for deaf children. In the UK, according to the British Association of Teachers of the Deaf (BATOD), 53 schools for deaf children closed between 1982 and 2017. There are currently 22 schools for deaf children remaining – a reduction in numbers of schools for deaf children of 70% over 35 years. In China, many schools for the deaf have either closed down or merged with schools for the blind or schools for children with autism or additional special educational needs. In Hong Kong, there is only 1 deaf school left catering to around 60–70 deaf students of all grade levels, and many of them have other special needs in addition to deafness.

Another challenge lies in how research findings can be used to impact and influence effective teaching practices in deaf education. Adam (2015) argues that research focusing on sign languages and Deaf communities should always have a public engagement element. In terms of informing the society about ways to educate deaf children, systematic research investigating the linguistic processes of how deaf children acquire sign language alongside a spoken language has just emerged recently (Lillo-Martin et al., 2016; Tang & Li, 2018). This kind of research is necessary because it would enable ToDs to access the most up to date research findings relating to the interaction between sign language and spoken language in order to support them to improve their teaching practices in sign bilingual settings.

Knoors and Marschark (2012) further commented that sign bilingual education remains as a strong theoretical assumption because the lack of robust empirical evidence makes it difficult to evaluate the effectiveness of sign bilingual education in bolstering literacy development and academic outcomes of deaf children. Also, their concern over quality sign language input in sign bilingual education stems from the fact that a majority of ToDs are hearing and adult learners of sign language, and that hearing parents of deaf children typically have little or no previous knowledge of sign language or contact with the Deaf community. In other words, the quantity and quality of sign language input to these children is bound to be different when compared with deaf children born to Deaf parents.

In contrast, in situations where neonatal screening and advanced assistive hearing technology are increasingly prominent, an increasing body of evidence is emerging showing that deaf children who are implanted or aided early have improved access to hearing and potential to develop speech. Based on these observations, Knoors and Marschark (2012) propose to re-examine the conditions for a bilingual language policy and suggest that more consideration should be given to the role of sign-supported speech or simultaneous communication in deaf children's language development and education. These issues remain controversial, especially from a linguistic point of view. For instance, Lund (2016) did not find any evidence that implanted children have the same vocabulary knowledge as their same-age peers, and Lund et al. (2014) did not find any correlation between vocabulary knowledge and implanted children's phonological awareness.

4.   Emerging developments in deaf education

4.1   Co-enrollment as a new form of sign bilingual education in mainstream education

One big challenge in light of this shift of educational context is the question of whether there is still a role and use of sign language for deaf children in mainstream education, as they are more oriented towards learning speech. Nevertheless, in countries where deaf children's rights are protected, they are able to access a mainstream curriculum through sign language, using sign interpreters or peripatetic ToDs. Yet, the effective inclusion of deaf children in mainstream schools does present some other challenges – particularly the social integration of deaf children with their peers (McKee, 2008). One solution to this challenge has been to combine sign bilingualism with co-enrollment, a relatively new concept that emphasizes co-learning between a critical mass of deaf and hearing students, and co-teaching between a hearing teacher who can sign and a Deaf signing teacher (Kirchner,

1994; Yiu et al., in press). Originating from the Tripod Program in the US, co-enrollment programmes have spread to the Netherlands (Hermans et al., 2014) and Spain (Martin, Balanzategui, & Morgan, 2014) in Europe. Both programmes reported gains in vocabulary development in a sign language and a spoken language. Additionally, for the programme in Madrid, researchers observed good social-emotional development among the deaf children and a shift from early sign language dominance to spoken language dominance. In Asia, Hong Kong has been trialling this approach since 2006, proposing that barriers of communication in mainstream classrooms can be alleviated and inclusion enhanced when both deaf and hearing children are nurtured to become bimodal bilinguals. The Sign Bilingualism and Co-enrollment in Education Programme (SLCO Programme) was launched at a kindergarten in 2006, annually moving up a grade level until currently reaching Grade 12 of secondary education. So far, positive outcomes have been documented in terms of positive language growth and correlations between HKSL, written Chinese and Cantonese (Tang et al., 2014); positive social integration (Yiu & Tang, 2014); and early metalinguistic differentiation between the signing varieties that represent either the grammar of HKSL or Cantonese / written Chinese (Tang et al., 2015). When the SLCO Programme was set up in Hong Kong, Bencie Woll was invited to serve as one of the external experts. In her 2010 interim report, she states, "The integrated approach to bilingualism which is at the heart of the project is to be commended and contrasts favourably both with bilingual programmes in other countries which seek to artificially separate the use of spoken and sign language and only teach sign language first, and with programmes in which inclusion in mainstream education without consideration of the individual child is seen as the answer for all deaf children. The evidence that learning HKSL does not negatively impact on spoken language development needs to be disseminated as widely as possible in Hong Kong."

The positive impact of the SLCO Programme has encouraged some neighbouring countries to develop similar co-enrollment programmes in pre-school and primary education. In Taiwan, Hsing (2016) summarizes the attempts by various researchers and educators to develop co-enrollment programmes primarily in pre-school education in different parts of Taiwan. Other countries and cities in Asia that have started co-enrollment programmes are Singapore,[5] Macau,[6] as well as some deaf schools in China. In a sense, co-enrollment may be seen as a reaction towards the lack of sign language, Deaf teachers and Deaf peer support in mainstream education, although access to a full curriculum is ensured. However, a

5. <http://www.straitstimes.com/singapore/education/mayflower-primary-to-take-in-deaf-pupils>

6. <http://www.exmoo.com/article/30779.html>

better understanding of how sign language and spoken language can work together in educating deaf children does require some fundamental research concerning language interactions in bilingual development.

4.2 Increasing diversity in deaf children's linguistic repertoire

The shifting context of deaf education suggests that deaf children nowadays may come from different learning environments, surrounded by a society that is becoming increasingly diverse and multilingual itself. That they are supported by increasingly sophisticated hearing technologies allowing them better access to speech albeit with different degrees of success also means that they represent a population of a diverse use of sign and spoken languages. This brings us back to the arena of the bilingual education literature. Simultaneously, the term 'translanguaging' has gained increasing currency in the wider field of multilingualism and bilingual education (Swanwick 2016). It presents a view of additive bilingualism where the acquisition of a second or additional language is seen as beneficial and not detrimental to the language user and the other languages in play. Swanwick (2016, 2017) argues that 'translanguaging' is particularly pertinent to deaf education where sign language competency has not been valued as an educational outcome. In this context, 'translanguaging' refers to the fluid use of sign, spoken and written language in the classroom by deaf learners and their teachers. It recognizes the diverse linguistic repertoires of deaf learners in their totality and moves away from defining language use purely in term of separate languages. This perspective of 'translanguaging' echoes recent findings of linguistic, neuroscience and cognitive psychology pointing to the advantage of being bimodal bilingual. In other words, 'translanguaging' is seen as a positive step towards understanding and enhancing bilingual deaf education provision where language policies rather than learner repertoire have tended to lead practice. In the UK, this trend of research has led to the development of a language planning teaching toolkit jointly developed by University of Leeds and practitioners from deaf schools and services in the Sign Bilingual Consortium in the UK aiming to provide strategies and resources to support ToDs and other professionals to deliver personalised language programmes for deaf multi-lingual learners (Swanwick et al., 2014).

4.3 Perception of language interaction as a natural outcome of bilingual development

Teaching practitioners have observed how deaf children produce the so-called 'non-standard' spoken language during their language acquisition process, and have suspected that this is related to the impact of learning sign language.

However, in child bilingual acquisition research, this phenomenon is referred to as 'crosslinguistic interactions' (Lillo-Martin et al., 2016) as a reflection on the processes involved in developing bimodal bilingualism or as 'bilingual co-activation' in psycholinguistics (Emmorey et al., 2015). In other words, language interaction is a natural outcome when children have knowledge of more than one grammar. There is plenty of evidence confirming that language interaction is amodal, which resonates an earlier argument by Cummins (2006) that transfer can occur at the conceptual, metalinguistic, linguistic and phonological levels, regardless of differences in modality.

For instance, recent years have seen a growing interest in the phenomenon of code blending by deaf and hearing children born of Deaf parents, that is, simultaneous use of sign language and spoken language in language production (van den Bogaerde, 2005 on NGT-Dutch; Branchini & Donati, 2016 on LIS-Italian, Fung & Tang, 2016 on HKSL-Cantonese; Lillo-Martin et al., 2016 on ASL-English). This rule-based linguistic behaviour is observed to follow the grammar of either language of the pair and reflect grammatical properties contributed by both languages, suggesting that bimodal bilinguals have at their disposal not one but two developing grammars in the acquisition process. Tang and Li (2018) argue that even for deaf children of hearing parents who are exposed to sign language later than spoken language, early exposure to sign language in a co-enrollment environment allows consistent sign language input to support early development of bimodal bilingualism as well as linguistic differentiation. (i.e. HKSL and Cantonese). They argue that crosslinguistic interaction and subsequent differentiation lay the foundation of language knowledge of deaf children, ensuring a more enriched linguistic repertoire in their performance.

5. Sign bilingual education in the future

Having summarized the history of sign bilingual education, the challenges and issues surrounding the growing demand of today's technological and bilingual/multilingual society and how it impacts the philosophy of deaf education, amid the growing interest in research of bimodal bilingualism and bilingual advantage, we will propose the following strategies for ensuring and consolidating high quality sign bilingual education in the future.

5.1 Educational environment

The shifting context of deaf education from specialist schools for the deaf to mainstream may be seen as an impetus for change as part and parcel of the evolution of sign bilingual education. Given the premise that natural languages transcend modality and are acquirable by humans, children and adults alike, sign language can potentially yield significant advantages to deaf children. Some studies discussed above have already shown that it supports them to access a full curriculum and develop spoken language within the general framework of bimodal bilingualism. Co-enrollment also creates and expands the signing community at school, as hearing children supported by Deaf teachers are also acquiring sign language at a young age and becoming bimodal bilingual, which enables them to communicate with deaf children as peers without barriers and with Deaf members of the Deaf community at large. Co-enrollment also requires inclusiveness in pedagogy; in other words, Deaf and hearing teachers collaborate effectively and develop flexible and dynamic approaches towards working with sign and spoken languages – in the classroom context to support both deaf and hearing children. Nevertheless, schools for the deaf still have an important role as part of the continuum of sign bilingual education provision because of the ToDs' specialist knowledge, skills, pedagogy and engagement in research. As centres of excellence, they can become trainers for mainstream teachers and provide advice, guidance and training on effective sign bilingual teaching practices, Deaf studies, deaf students' language development and appropriate educational resources to practitioners in mainstream settings. Also, there are still many deaf children who are unable to benefit from mainstream education, and they require a more specialised and personalised curriculum that only schools for the deaf can provide.

Professional training in sign bilingual education
Although technology and philosophy of education has changed rapidly during the last few decades, the sign bilingual approach ensures that sign language remains a valuable element in deaf education and is very much a part of the continuum of educational provision in elementary education. This is both in terms of the development of practice and of an educational philosophy that is open to new research evidence and developments at the global level. As we have seen, sign bilingual education is in a continual state of evolution so practitioners need to be informed of up-to-date research findings in order to continue to adapt their teaching to maximize deaf children's potential. Therefore, the training of practitioners, particularly Deaf people, who are becoming increasingly involved in the education process, becomes a necessity. Ongoing sign language training to improve the signing proficiency of hearing practitioners who teach deaf children in either deaf school or mainstream school setting is called for to ensure quality of instruction, especially the awareness of specialist teaching skills that bridge deaf children's awareness about sign and spoken/written languages for their ultimate literacy development (Wauters & de Klerk, 2014).

5.2   Involvement of deaf ToDs

We would argue it is important to employ increasing numbers of Deaf people in schools and services. In addition to their serving as linguistic role models, they should also be fully involved in developing a curriculum to teach deaf children about their Deaf identity, sign language, culture and heritage. In the UK, the Deaf Studies Working Group was established in 1999 and published a Deaf Studies Curriculum, which has been adopted by most bilingual deaf schools and services across the UK. They are currently collaborating on the development of a BSL linguistics curriculum for the UK. In Australia, the Australian Curriculum, Assessment and Reporting Authority (ACARA) officially published the first national curriculum for AUSLAN in August 2017. The SLCO Programme of Hong Kong has resulted in some Deaf ToDs graduating with a Bachelor's degree in special education, which is unprecedented in the history of HK's deaf education. The Chinese University of Hong Kong will also launched a Bachelor of Arts programme in Bimodal Bilingual Studies in 2019 to nurture more ToDs proficient in HKSL. At the SLCO schools, in addition to classroom teaching, Deaf ToDs are responsible for teaching HKSL to the stakeholders and organizing a Deaf festival for the whole school every year in order to inculcate Deaf awareness in a mainstream school environment.

Involvement of Deaf ToDs also ensures that deaf children grow up surrounded by Deaf social role models and achieve a sense of 'belonging' at home, at school and in the wider community. This supports them to develop strong emotional bonds, a sense of positive well-being, and a better understanding of social norms. ToDs also connect the deaf children back to the Deaf community so that, in time, they develop a greater choice and flexibility to move between their deaf and hearing friendship groups with confidence and success.

5.3   Sign language and parents

To avoid compromising communication between the parents and deaf children, it is important to support parents through sign language training because they need sign language to communicate with their children at an appropriate level from the earliest age possible. In some programmes in the UK, Deaf staff teach BSL in the home to parents and extended family. Deaf schools and resource centres that are co-located with mainstream schools also run BSL courses for the staff, hearing children and their families. In Hong Kong, a non-government organization was set up in 2017 to promote early bimodal bilingualism for deaf and hearing children.[7]

---

7. The SLCO Community Resources <http://www.slco.org.hk/en/index.php>

5.4 The nature of sign-supported speech in sign bilingual programmes

Knoors and Marschark (2012) argued for more consideration be given to "sign-supported speech (SSS)" in the education of deaf children, which is picked up by Swanwick (2016) as a natural form of linguistic behaviour when deaf and hearing bimodal bilinguals interact with each other especially in the classroom context. However, one should not lose sight of the central tenet of sign bilingual education now boosted by findings of recent sign linguistic research. Practitioners need to be made aware that SSS has a secondary though supportive role, while primacy still goes to natural sign language as a language of instruction and communication in sign bilingual programmes. Nevertheless, given the diverse linguistic repertoires of deaf students nowadays, SSS may sometimes serve to open up communication to certain groups of deaf and hearing children who are at different stages of bilingual development themselves. Indeed, in the SLCO Programme of Hong Kong, it is the deaf students who try to accommodate to the learning needs of their hearing peers by resorting to SSS when communicating with them at the initial stage of their HKSL development while these deaf students use HKSL among themselves. Realistically, SSS is there to stay because it represents one of the common phenomena of crosslinguistic interaction manifesting itself through a continuum of signing varieties with greater or lesser degrees of manually coded spoken language. However, practitioners should be trained to be aware of this distinction between natural sign language and SSS, and adopt appropriate pedagogical strategies to help students differentiate the signing systems.

5.5 International movement towards promoting the linguistic status of sign language and its role in deaf children's education

At this juncture, it is worth pointing out that the CRPD,[8] adopted in 2006, goes some way in recognising the cultural and linguistic identities of Deaf communities and sign languages around the world. Murray et al. (2018) discuss how the CRPD signifies a shift from the medical model of disability to the social model (2018: 39). Article 2 recognises in its definition of language that sign language and spoken language are of equal status, and Article 24 refers to the right to use sign language in education.[9] In 2018, April, the CRPD committee further commented that "the lack of sign language learning environments, deaf peers, Deaf adult

---

8. <https://www.un.org/development/desa/disabilities/convention-on-the-rights-of-persons-with-disabilities.html>

9. Article 24 (3) (c) states: "education of persons, and in particular, children who are blind, deaf or deafblind, is delivered in the most appropriate languages and modes and means of

role models and teachers qualified in sign language is considered discriminatory toward deaf children".[10] In response to this comment, The World Federation of the Deaf (WFD) in June 2018 announced a Position Paper on Inclusion in Education[11] in which they argued that effective inclusive education for deaf students include high-quality deaf schools which employ many Deaf ToDs to support deaf students in mainstream education. Another form of high-quality inclusive education is co-enrolment "where a team of deaf and hearing teachers provide simultaneous instruction in sign language and spoken language to classrooms of deaf and hearing students". Whichever form of co-enrollment one adopts, importance is attached to deaf students learning sign language, and Deaf teachers employed on an equal basis to their hearing colleagues. Clearly such international movements will cast a significantly positive impact on bringing sign language and Deaf ToDs back to deaf education in different settings.

6. Conclusion

In this chapter, we have offered an overview of sign bilingual education in countries that we are familiar with, highlighting prominent but common themes such as language of instruction, impacts of technological advances and changing educational contexts. We have also explored the challenges to the sign bilingual this approach in the 21st century and how these have triggered new developments to accommodate sign bilingual education in different educational settings. We argue that more research is necessary to better understand how deaf children acquire, process and use sign language and spoken language. At the practical level, more research is needed on literacy and wider educational attainment of deaf children in order to inform practitioners about the optimum conditions for developing effective sign bilingual practices across different educational contexts. Sign bilingual education is no longer a theoretical assumption it is established, growing and evolving in many parts of the world, and hopefully will continue to stimulate positive developments into the next decades and beyond.

---

communication for the individual, and in environments which maximise academic and social development."

10. <https://wfdeaf.org/news/wfds-input-results-crpd-committee-acknowledgement-deaf-children-must-full-accessibility-schools-sign-language/>

11. <http://wfdeaf.org/news/resources/5-june-2018-wfd-position-paper-inclusive-education/>

Acknowledgment

We would like to acknowledge the comments and contributions made by Ruth Swanwick, School of Education, University of Leeds, UK, on the initial drafts of this paper.

References

Adam, R. (2015). Public engagement with the Deaf Community. In E. Orfanidou, B. Woll, & G. Morgan (Eds.), *Guides to research methods in language and linguistics. The Blackwell guide to research methods in sign language studies* (pp. 41–52). Hoboken NJ: Wiley Blackwell.

Ainscow, M. (2005). Developing inclusive education systems: What are the levers for change? *Journal of Educational Change* 6, 109–124.   https://doi.org/10.1007/s10833-005-1298-4

Auslan/English Bilingual Education: A survey of Australian programs. (2001). Report by Hearing Impairment Services, West Group Districts, South Australia.

Branchini, C., & Donati, C. (2016). Assessing lexicalism through bimodal eyes. *Glossa: A Journal of General Linguistics* 1, 1–30. doi: https://doi.org/10.5334/gjgl.29

Burchett, J. H. (1964). *Utmost for the highest: The story of the Victorian School for Deaf children.* Melbourne: Hall's Book Stall.

Conrad, R. (1979). *The deaf school child: Language and cognitive function.* London: Harper Row.

Cummins, J. (2006). The relationship between American Sign Language proficiency and English academic development: A review of the research. Paper presented at the Workshop Challenges, Opportunities, and Choices in Education Minority Group Students, October, 2006, Hamar University College, Norway.

Carty, B. M. (2004). *Managing their own affairs: The Australian deaf community during the 1920s and 1930s* (Unpublished doctoral dissertation). Griffith University.

CRIDE. (2011). *Report on 2011 survey on educational provision for deaf children in England.* <www.ndcs.org.uk/CRIDE>

CRIDE. (2017). *Report on 2017 (UK-wide summary) survey on educational provision for deaf children.* <www.ndcs.org.uk/CRIDE>

Emmorey, K., Giezen, M. R., & Gollan, T. H. (2015). Psycholinguistic, cognitive, and neural implications of bimodal bilingual. *Bilingualism: Language and Cognition* 19, 223–242. https://doi.org/10.1017/S1366728915000085.

Fung, C. H.-M., & Tang, G. (2016). Code-blending of functional heads in Hong Kong Sign Language and Cantonese: A case study. *Bilingualism: Language and Cognition* 19(4): 754–781. https://doi.org/10.1017/S1366728915000747.

Geers, A. E., Mitchell, C. M., Warner-Czyz, A., Wang, N-Y., Eisenberg, L. S., & CDaCI Investigative Team. (2017). Early sign language exposure and cochlear implantation benefits. *Pediatrics* 140(1), e20163489.   https://doi.org/10.1542/peds.2016-3489

Hermans, D., de Klerk, A., Wauters, L., & Knoors, H. (2014). The Twinschool: A co-enrollment program in Netherlands. In M. Marschark, G. Tang, & H. Knoors (Eds.), *Bilingualism and bilingual deaf education* (pp. 396–323). New York, NY: Oxford University Press. https://doi.org/10.1093/acprof:oso/9780199371815.003.0016

Hermans, D., Ormel, E., & Knoors, H. (2010). On the relation between the signing and reading skills of deaf bilinguals. *International Journal of Bilingual Education and Bilingualism* 13, 187–199. https://doi.org/10.1080/3670050903474093

Hettiarachchi, S., de Silva, M. D., Wijesinghe, T., Susantha, B., Amila, G., Sarani, P., &Rasak, M. (in press). 'Free but not fair': A critical review of access to equal and equitable education to deaf children in Sri Lanka. In M. Marschark & H. Knoors (Eds.), *Deaf education in developing countries*. Oxford: Oxford University Press.

Hsing, M.-H. (2016). 國外聽障教育手語雙語模色考察建議 (Models of sign bilingual education in overseas countries: A survey report and recommendations). Manuscript.

Humphries, T., Kushalnagar, P., Mathur, G., Napoli, D. J., Padden, C., & Rathman, C. (2014). Ensuring language acquisition for deaf children: What linguistics can do. *Language* 90, e31–e52. http://dx.doi.org/10.1353/lan.2014.0036. https://doi.org/10.1353/lan.2014.0036

Kirchner, C. J. (1994). Co-enrollment as an inclusion model. *American Annals of the Deaf* 139(2): 163–164. https://doi.org/10.1353/aad.2012.0187

Johnston T., & Schembri, A. (2007). *Australian Sign Language (Auslan): An introduction to sign language linguistics*. Cambridge: Cambridge University Press. https://doi.org/10.1017/CBO9780511607479

Jhang, se-Eun. (2015). Notes on Korean Sign Language. In C. Lee, S. B. Greg, & Y. Kim (Eds.), *The handbook of East Asian psycholinguistics, Vol. III: Korean* (pp. 361–378). Cambridge: Cambridge University Press.

Knoors, H. & Marschark, M. (2012). Language planning for the 21st century: Revisiting bilingual language policy for deaf children. *Journal of Deaf Studies and Deaf Education* 17(3): 291–305. https://doi.org/10.1093/deafed/ens018

Lillo-Martin, D., de Quadros, R. M., & Chen-Pichler, D. (2016). The development of bimodal bilingualism: Implications for linguistics theory. *Linguistic Approaches to Bilingualism* 6, 719–755. https://doi.org/10.1075/lab.6.6.01lil

Lund, E. (2016). Vocabulary knowledge of children with cochlear implants: A meta-analysis. *Journal of Deaf Studies and Deaf Education* 21(2): 107–121. https://doi.org/10.1093/deafed/env060

Lund, E., Werfel, K. E., & Schuele, C. M. (2014). Phonological awareness and vocabulary performance of monolingual and bilingual preschool children with hearing loss. *Child Language Teaching and Therapy* 31(12): 85–100.

Napoli, D. J., Mellon, N. K., Niparko, J. K., Rathmann, C., Mathur, G., Humphries, T., Handley, T., Scambler, S., & Lantos, H. D. (2015). Should all deaf children learn sign language? *Paediatrics* 136(1), 170–176. https://doi.org/10.1542/peds.2014-1632

Martin, M. P., Balanzategui, M. V., & Morgan, G. (2014). Sign bilingual and co-enrollment education for children with cochlear implants in Madrid, Spain. In M. Marschark, G. Tang, & H. Knoors (Eds.), *Bilingualism and bilingual deaf education* (pp. 368–395). New York, NY: Oxford University Press. https://doi.org/10.1093/acprof:oso/9780199371815.003.0015

Mayer, C., & Leigh, G. (2010). The changing context for sign bilingual education programs: Issues in language and the development of literacy. *International Journal of Bilingual Education and Bilingualism* 13(2), 175–186. <http://www.tanfonline.com/loi/rbeb20> https://doi.org/10.1080/13670050903474085

McKee, R. L. (2008). 'As one deaf person to another': Deaf paraprofessionals in mainstream schools. *Deaf Worlds* 21(1), 1–48.

Murray, J. J., Snoddon, K., De Meulder, M., & Underwood, K. (2018). Intersectional inclusion for deaf learners: Moving beyond General Comment #4 on Article 24 of the United Nations Convention on the Rights of Persons with Disabilities. *International Journal of Inclusive Education*. https://doi.org/10.1080/13603116.2018.1482013.

Plaza-Pust, C. (2012). Deaf education and bilingualism. In R. Pfau, M. Steinbach, & B. Woll. (Eds.), *Handbook on sign language* (pp. 949–979). Berlin: Mouton de Gruyter. https://doi.org/10.1515/9783110261325.949

Pickersgill, M., & Gregory, S. (1998). *Sign bilingualism: A model.* Adept Press, Middx: LASER.

Power, M. R., Power, D., & Horstmanshof, L. (2007). Deaf people communicating via SMS, TTY, relay service, fax, and computers in Australia. *Journal of Deaf Studies and Deaf Education* 12(1), 80–92. https://doi.org/10.1093/deafed/enl016

Special Educational Needs and Disability (SEND) Code of Practice: 0–25 years: Statutory guidance for organisations which work with and support children and young people who have special educational needs or disabilities. (2015). Published by Department of Education and Department of Health, UK Government, January 2015.

Swanwick, R., Simpson, K., & Salter, J. (2014). *Language planning in deaf education: Guidance for practitioners by practitioners teacher toolkit.* Leeds: NatSIP, University of Leeds, SBC and BSL coalition.

Swanwick, R. (2016). *Languages and languaging in deaf education: A framework for pedagogy.* New York, NY: Oxford University Press.

Swanwick, R. (2017). Translanguaging, learning and teaching in deaf education. *International Journal of Multilingualism* 14(3), 233–249. https://doi.org/10.1080/14790718.2017.1315808

Sze, F., Lo, C., Lo, L., & Chu, K. (2013). Historical development of Hong Kong Sign Language. *Sign Language Studies* 13(2), 155–185. https://doi.org/10.1353/sls.2013.0002

Tang, G., Chan, T., & Chan, D. (2006). Linguistic comprehension of natural sign language and simultaneous communication by deaf students: An experiment. Paper presented at *International Conference on Special Education*, Centre for Advancement in Special Education, June, The University of Hong Kong, Hong Kong.

Tang, G., Lam, S., & Yiu, C. (2014). Language development of deaf children in a sign bilingual and co-enrollment environment. In M. Marschark, G. Tang, & H. Knoors (Eds.), *Bilingualism and bilingual deaf education* (pp. 313–342). Oxford: Oxford University Press. https://doi.org/10.1093/acprof:oso/9780199371815.003.0013

Tang, G., Yiu, C., & Lam, S. (2015). Awareness of Hong Kong Sign Language and manually coded Chinese by deaf students. In H. Knoors & M. Marschark (Eds.), *Educating deaf learners: Creating a global evidence base* (pp. 117–148). Oxford: Oxford University Press. https://doi.org/10.1093/acprof:oso/9780190215194.003.0006

Tang, G., & Li, J. (2018). Acquisition of classifier constructions in HKSL by bimodal bilingual deaf children of hearing parents. *Frontiers in Psychology* 9, 1148. https://doi.org/10.3389/fpsyg.2018.01148.

Van den Bogaerde, B., & Baker, A. (2005). Code mixing in mother–child interaction in deaf families. *Sign Language & Linguistics* 8(1-2), 153–176. https://doi.org/10.1075/sll.8.1-2.08bog

Wauters, L. & de Klerk, A. (2014). Improving reading instruction to deaf and hard-of-hearing students. In M. Marschark, G. Tang, & H. Knoors (Eds.), *Bilingualism and bilingual deaf education* (pp. 368–395). New York, NY: Oxford University Press. https://doi.org/10.1093/acprof:oso/9780199371815.003.0010

Wheeler, A., Archbold, S., Gregory, S., & Skipp, A. (2007). Cochlear implants: The young people's perspective. *Journal of Deaf Studies and Deaf Education* 12(3), 303–316. https://doi.org/10.1093/deafed/enm018

Woodward, J., & Nguyen, H. T. (2012). Where sign language studies had led us in forty years: Opening high school and university education for deaf people in Vietnam through sign language analysis, teaching and interpretation. *Sign Language Studies* 13(1), 19–36. https://doi.org/10.1353/sls.2012.0023

Wu, A., Shen, Y. L., Zhang, N. S., & Chu, C. Y. (Eds.). (2005). 双语聋教育的理论与实践 (Practical and Theoretical Issues in Bilingual Education of the Deaf). Beijing: Huaxia.

Wu, L. (2008). 联合国儿童基金会聋儿双语双文化项目-中期评估报告 (UNICEF Bilingual-Bicultural Education for Deaf and Hard-of-Hearing children in China – Interim Evaluation Report).

Yang, J.-H. (2008). Sign language and oral/written language in deaf education in China. In C. Plaza-Pust & E. Morales-López (Eds.), *Sign bilingualism* (pp. 297–332). Amsterdam: John Benjamins. https://doi.org/10.1075/sibil.38.13yan

Yiu, C. K-M., & Tang, G. (2014). Social integration of deaf and hard-of-hearing students in a sign bilingual and co-enrollment environment. In M. Marschark, G. Tang, & H. Knoors (Eds.), *Bilingualism and bilingual deaf education* (pp. 342–367). Oxford: Oxford University Press. https://doi.org/10.1093/acprof:oso/9780199371815.003.0014

Yiu, C. K-M, Tang, G., & Ho, C. C-M. (in press). Essential ingredients for sign bilingualism and co-enrollment education in the Hong Kong context. In M. Marschark, H. Knoors, & S. Antia (Eds.), *Co-enrollment education for deaf and hard-of-hearing learners*. Oxford: Oxford University Press.

Past, present and future?

Ruth Campbell

Fifteen years ago, Bencie Woll, Gary Morgan, Gabriella Vigliocco and myself faced a panel of experts from the UK Economic and Social Science Research Council (ESRC) in a London conference room. We were being assessed for funding for a proposal for a research centre on deafness. 'Deafness …', we proposed '… offers an exciting model for approaching questions on language – its origins, development and processes …'. The panel's questions were incisive and probing. Panel members wondered how studies of sign language in deaf people could illuminate the nature of language and language processing. They pointed out that the numbers of people we planned to work with – primarily prelingually deaf people who had acquired a sign language from deaf carers and who were members of a deaf community, often educated at schools for the deaf – were relatively small. They reminded us that early hearing loss was being aggressively and effectively treated with neonatal testing. Advances in hearing aid (especially cochlear implant) and genetic technologies, alongside the successes achieved by mass vaccination for rubella and other infections in infancy, meant that the target population we planned to work with was not only small, but dwindling. While deafness may constitute a 'special case' in understanding language, its relevance to issues concerning language and language processing may be limited.

We did our best to counter this argument. Our plans, we pointed out, took full cognizance of the heterogeneity of deafness: we would explore language processing in people for whom BSL may not have been acquired early within a deaf culture; we would investigate how language processing may develop when speech was processed primarily by sight (speechreading) rather than by ear. We pointed out that the recent UK government 'Foresight' project to identify priority issues for scientific study had specifically indicated '… the investigation of features common to how the brain processes spoken language and sign language (SL) as one of six key questions facing researchers in language …' https://assets.publishing.service.gov.uk/government/uploads/system/uploads/attachment_data/file/300857/03-1336-cognitive-systems-overview.pdf. We assured the panel that

https://doi.org/10.1075/tilar.25.aft

our various disciplines of experimental, developmental and neuropsychology, psycholinguistics and linguistics meant that we would be able, as a team, to bring a special focus to the work.

Above all, with Bencie as the project Director, we had the leading scholar whose reputation in sign language research, and with the Deaf community, was second to none. We convinced the panel that our team – and our team in collaboration with researchers elsewhere, could develop a programme of research that would ensure that UK research in deafness and sign language would be at the forefront of top-rank international research.

Our arguments were accepted and DCAL was born. Now, 15 years on, the role of the study of sign languages in broader explorations of the study of language is well attested. Google Scholar searches for 'sign language' show 213,000 citations in the period 1995–2005, in comparison to a three-fold increase to 637,000 in 2005–2015. For 'sign language, brain' the citation figures are 298,000 in the period 1995–2005, in comparison to an almost four-fold increase to 1,140,000 in 2005–2015. A search for 'deaf studies' gave 91,600 in 1995–2005 as compared to 143,000 in 2005–2015.

Deafness research is firmly on the map as far as academic scholarship is concerned. What has happened to deafness research in these fifteen years – and where is it going? Even before meeting Bencie in 1994, I was struck by the lack of engagement of the academic disciplines around cognitive language science with the varieties of experience that were evident in deaf people. Language Sciences were construed almost exclusively in terms of heard speech. Where sign languages and deafness had entered the picture they were often seen as marginal, even exotic (Sacks, 1989). In child development, the majority of studies involving deaf children were focused on their pesky inability to reach 'appropriate reading levels' despite age-appropriate non-verbal intelligence (I had done several experiments in this field!). The study of communication in deaf people existed in an academic 'ghetto'; benign, perhaps, but at a remove from the mainstream of scientific research. Deafness research was seen as the province of clinical and professional specialists, largely tasked with bringing scientific ideas, often based on studies of hearing, non-signing people, to the clinic (usually the audiology clinic) or the educational setting (schools for the deaf).

Is this still the case? Has work in the clinic become better informed by research based on language processing in deaf people? Have the academic disciplines around language and communication become more accepting of deafness and deaf-related insights into language and cognition? Thanks to Bencie's pioneering exposition of BSL structure, and her key role in developing instruments for assessing sign language skills, sophisticated tests appropriate for assessing language skills in British deaf populations can now be used to inform the clinic and the school setting (Herman et al., 2004; Vinson, Cormier, Denmark, Schembri, & Vigliocco,

2008). Deaf people with clinical conditions can now be appropriately investigated (Atkinson, Denmark, Marshall, Mummery, & Woll, 2015). Tests developed through DCAL for BSL users can be models for users of other sign languages (Haug & Mann, 2008). The DCAL-based work on developing a representative corpus of BSL has meant that language change and BSL language variation in the UK can inform work in the clinic (Stamp et al., 2014). Within DCAL we were able to support and advance deaf researchers' skills, so that their insights would be properly embedded in findings, and their academic careers could advance effectively.

It would be satisfying to report that work in the academy had taken a similar turn and accommodated insights from deafness into mainstream language science. To some extent this has been the case. There has been a shift in the dynamic that drives language research. For example, issues around iconicity in both spoken and signed language are being explored more fully (Perniss, Thompson, & Vigliocco, 2010; Perniss & Vigliocco, 2014). Speech and language processing takes more account of the impact of modalities other than auditory – the perception of spoken language is accepted to have visual aspects, as in speechreading (Campbell, MacSweeney, & Waters, 2008) and modality issues are now considered along with linguistic ones. Largely thanks to earlier insights into the formal grammatical aspects of sign language (Stokoe, 2005), gesture and nonverbal behaviours accompanying speech have come to be explored within a broader linguistic and psycholinguistic framework (Goldin Meadow, 2003).

In the present collection, the chapters by Morgan, by Harris and Clibbens, and by Baker and Van den Bogaerde, show how the experiences of deaf children and their carers clarify necessary and sufficient conditions for acquiring effective communication in language whether spoken or signed. It remains the case, however, that these studies were needed to correct under-informed assumptions about – for instance – developmental lags in deaf children's 'theory of mind' skills (Morgan, Jones & Botting, this volume).

In neuroscience, too, we have had to correct misinterpretations concerning neuroplasticity for language. Some of the most profound misunderstandings reflect the fact that much historical research was based on studies of non-linguistic deaf animals, leading to an emphasis on auditory, rather than language and communication rehabilitation. Such assumptions can infiltrate the clinic (Campbell, MacSweeney, & Woll, 2014). Recent scholarly focus on commonalities and differences for signed and for spoken language structures may direct more thoughtful approaches in relation to brain imaging (Lillo-Martin & Gajewski, 2014).

Much more work remains to be done to explore the varieties of bimodal bilingualism – that is, to explore the neural circuits involved in language processing whether in speech or sign language – in deaf and in hearing populations. While DCAL and other research teams have made a start on this (Capek, Campbell, &

Woll, 2008; Emmorey, Giezen, & Gollan, 2016; Kovelman, Shalinsky, Berens, & Petitto, 2014; Olulade et al., 2016), the relative reliance on one or other language mode, and the age of acquisition of each language, require closer scrutiny. Here CoDA – hearing children of Deaf adults – will help clarify the picture. Greater left-hemisphere language lateralization can be observed in CoDA signers compared with hearing monolingual speakers (Gutierrez-Sigut et al., 2015), possibly reflecting the additional recruitment of left-parietal regions in articulating signs in space (and see Cardin et al.'s chapter). Not all CoDA use sign language – but could their brains nevertheless show any trace of early exposure to sign? CoDA infants' looking behavior to faces differs from that of hearing infants with hearing parents – presumably reflecting these prelingual infants' sensitivity to the communication patterns of their parents (Mercure et al., 2019; Mercure et al., 2018). And what of those bimodal bilinguals who acquire a sign language as a second language: a relatively large group of hearing people, often working as support workers with Deaf people or as sign language interpreters? Clarifying similarities and differences in neural as well as behavioural terms will flesh out current theorizing about how first and further languages are processed, and the role of modality of language in its acquisition and development.

Some of the deepest recent insights into language development come from studies of linguistic development in the large and relatively under-examined population of deaf children of hearing parents. As Morgan (Chapter 2) shows, such children lack not only hearing, but the common conditions for language learning – including adult language models. Thanks to the development of appropriate language tests, it is now clear that such delayed (sign-)language development leaves a lasting trace on cognitive, communicative and linguistic performance (MacSweeney, Waters, Brammer, Woll, & Goswami, 2008). Even when there seems, superficially, to be good accommodation to language, effects of late language learning (LLL) in deaf adults can remain in terms of neural structures and networks (Mayberry, Davenport, Roth, & Halgren, 2018).

The landscape of deafness itself has changed in these years. Around 80% of children born deaf in the USA are now thought to have cochlear implants (CI). In the preschool and school populations in the US and the UK, around half of all children with early deafness will have CI, and early CI has been shown to be beneficial in terms of the deaf child's speech-based skills and learning. Implantees occupy a relatively new zone in relation to deafness. These developments have implications for Deaf communities, and ethical quandaries abound (Humphries et al., 2012). Societal and professional changes follow (deaf schools close, audiological interventions increase).

Anthropologists have started to explore this phenomenon (Mauldin, 2016). For scholars of language and communication these societal changes are likely to interact with behavioral and neural descriptions, reflecting the impact of hearing restoration on this scale. Questions remain concerning the role of sign language for deaf children under these conditions (Geers et al., 2017; Hall, 2017). It should be noted that learning outcomes in implantees are variable (Harris, Terlektsi, & Kyle, 2017), while acknowledging that, following CI in infancy, many more deaf children will be able to thrive in hearing schools and settings (Geers, Tobey, Moog, & Brenner, 2008). The sources of this variability will need to be explored systematically: in behavioural studies it will be necessary to explore the extent to which language skills correlate not just with the use of CI, and the extent of auditory rehabilitation, but also the developmental and social milieu in which the person with CI was raised. Different neural signatures may be linked to these differences. One outstanding question must be the extent to which the cortical networks for language which have been identified for CoDA populations, and which can differ from those of deaf native signers, may appear in CI populations.

Can we claim, then, that the ESRC showed foresight in funding DCAL? Without doubt the impact of the research undertaken over the last fifteen years has meant that insights into language and communication from the perspective of deafness have become better integrated into language science scholarship, and will impact positively in deaf people's lives. We are well positioned now to explore how early cochlear implantation may impact on developing language and communication skills, their neural bases, and its impact on sign language users and communities. Above all, though, as this volume demonstrates, our communal enterprise in exploring language and communication in deafness has deepened our understanding of what it means to be born deaf, and has led us to consider more carefully how deaf people's experiences inform their and our lives.

References

Atkinson, J., Denmark, T., Marshall, J., Mummery, C., & Woll, B. (2015). Detecting cognitive impairment and dementia in deaf people: The British Sign Language Cognitive Screening Test. *Arch Clin Neuropsychol* 30(7), 694–711. Retrieved from: <https://www.ncbi.nlm.nih.gov/pubmed/26245349> https://doi.org/10.1093/arclin/acv042

Campbell, R., MacSweeney, M., & Waters, D. (2008). Sign language and the brain: A review. *J. Deaf Stud. Deaf Educ.*, 13(1), 3–20. Retrieved from: <http://www.ncbi.nlm.nih.gov/pubmed/17602162> https://doi.org/10.1093/deafed/enm035

Campbell, R., MacSweeney, M., & Woll, B. (2014). Cochlear implantation (CI) for prelingual deafness: The relevance of studies of brain organization and the role of first language acquisition in considering outcome success. *Front. Hum. Neurosci.*, 8, 834. Retrieved from: <https://www.ncbi.nlm.nih.gov/pubmed/25368567> https://doi.org/10.3389/fnhum.2014.00834

Capek, C., Campbell, R., & Woll, B. (2008). The bimodal bilingual brain: fMRI investigations concerning the cortical distribution and differentiation of signed language and speechreading. *Rivista di Psicolinguistica Applicata* VIII, 18.

Emmorey, K., Giezen, M. R., & Gollan, T. H. (2016). Psycholinguistic, cognitive, and neural implications of bimodal bilingualism. *Biling. (Camb Engl)* 19(2), 223–242. Retrieved from: <https://www.ncbi.nlm.nih.gov/pubmed/28804269> https://doi.org/10.1017/S1366728915000085

Geers, A., Tobey, E., Moog, J., & Brenner, C. (2008). Long-term outcomes of cochlear implantation in the preschool years: From elementary grades to high school. *Int. J. Audiol.*, 47(Suppl 2), S21–S30. Retrieved from: <https://www.ncbi.nlm.nih.gov/pubmed/19012109> https://doi.org/10.1080/14992020802339167

Geers, A. E., Mitchell, C. M., Warner-Czyz, A., Wang, N. Y., Eisenberg, L. S., & Team, C. I. (2017). Early sign language exposure and cochlear implantation benefits. *Pediatrics* 140(1). Retrieved from: <https://www.ncbi.nlm.nih.gov/pubmed/28759398> https://doi.org/10.1542/peds.2016-3489

Goldin Meadow, S. (2003). *The resilience of language: What gesture creation in deaf children can tell us about how all children learn language.* New York, NY: Psychology Press.

Gutierrez-Sigut, E., Daws, R., Payne, H., Blott, J., Marshall, C., & MacSweeney, M. (2015). Language lateralization of hearing native signers: A functional transcranial Doppler sonography (fTCD) study of speech and sign production. *Brain Lang.*, 151, 23–34. Retrieved from: <https://www.ncbi.nlm.nih.gov/pubmed/26605960> https://doi.org/10.1016/j.bandl.2015.10.006

Hall, W. C. (2017). What you don't know can hurt you: The risk of language deprivation by impairing sign language development in deaf children. *Matern. Child Health J.*, 21(5), 961–965. Retrieved from: <https://www.ncbi.nlm.nih.gov/pubmed/28185206> https://doi.org/10.1007/s10995-017-2287-y

Harris, M., Terlektsi, E., & Kyle, F. E. (2017). Literacy outcomes for Primary School children who are deaf and hard of hearing: A cohort comparison study. *J. Speech Lang. Hear. Res.*, 60(3), 701–711. Retrieved from: <https://www.ncbi.nlm.nih.gov/pubmed/28241207> https://doi.org/10.1044/2016_JSLHR-H-15-0403

Haug, T., & Mann, W. (2008). Adapting tests of sign language assessment for other sign languages--a review of linguistic, cultural, and psychometric problems. *J. Deaf Stud. Deaf Educ.*, 13(1), 138–147. Retrieved from <https://www.ncbi.nlm.nih.gov/pubmed/17569751> https://doi.org/10.1093/deafed/enm027

Herman, R., Grove, N., Holmes, G., Morgan, G., Sutherland, H., & Woll, B. (2004). *Assessing BSL Development:Production Test.* [Narrative production test]. London.

Humphries, T., Kushalnagar, P., Mathur, G., Napoli, D. J., Padden, C., Rathmann, C., & Smith, S. R. (2012). Language acquisition for deaf children: Reducing the harms of zero tolerance to the use of alternative approaches. *Harm Reduct. J.*, 9(1), 16. Retrieved from: <http://www.ncbi.nlm.nih.gov/pubmed/22472091> https://doi.org/10.1186/1477-7517-9-16

Kovelman, I., Shalinsky, M. H., Berens, M. S., & Petitto, L. A. (2014). Words in the bilingual brain: an fNIRS brain imaging investigation of lexical processing in sign-speech bimodal bilinguals. *Front. Hum. Neurosci.*, 8, 606. Retrieved from: <http://www.ncbi.nlm.nih.gov/pubmed/25191247> https://doi.org/10.3389/fnhum.2014.00606

Lillo-Martin, D. C., & Gajewski, J. (2014). One grammar or two? Sign languages and the nature of human language. *Wiley Interdiscip. Rev. Cogn. Sci.*, 5(4), 387–401. Retrieved from: <https://www.ncbi.nlm.nih.gov/pubmed/25013534> https://doi.org/10.1002/wcs.1297

MacSweeney, M., Waters, D., Brammer, M. J., Woll, B., & Goswami, U. (2008). Phonological processing in deaf signers and the impact of age of first language acquisition. *Neuroimage* 40(3), 1369–1379. Retrieved from: <http://www.ncbi.nlm.nih.gov/pubmed/18282770>. https://doi.org/10.1016/j.neuroimage.2007.12.047

Mauldin, L. (2016). *Made to hear: Cochlear implants and raising deaf children*. Minneapolis, MN: University of Minnesota Press.

Mayberry, R. I., Davenport, T., Roth, A., & Halgren, E. (2018). Neurolinguistic processing when the brain matures without language. *Cortex* 99, 390–403. Retrieved from: <https://www.ncbi.nlm.nih.gov/pubmed/29406150> https://doi.org/10.1016/j.cortex.2017.12.011

Mercure, E., Kushnerenko, E., Goldberg, L., Bowden-Howl, H., Coulson, K., Johnson, M. H., & MacSweeney, M. (2019). Language experience influences audiovisual speech integration in unimodal and bimodal bilingual infants. *Dev. Sci.*, 22(1), e12701. Retrieved from: <https://www.ncbi.nlm.nih.gov/pubmed/30014580> https://doi.org/10.1111/desc.12701

Mercure, E., Quiroz, I., Goldberg, L., Bowden-Howl, H., Coulson, K., Gliga, T., … MacSweeney, M. (2018). Impact of language experience on attention to faces in infancy: Evidence from unimodal and bimodal bilingual infants. *Front. Psychol.*, 9, 1943. Retrieved from: <https://www.ncbi.nlm.nih.gov/pubmed/30459671> https://doi.org/10.3389/fpsyg.2018.01943

Olulade, O. A., Jamal, N. I., Koo, D. S., Perfetti, C. A., LaSasso, C., & Eden, G. F. (2016). Neuroanatomical evidence in support of the bilingual advantage theory. *Cereb. Cortex* 26(7), 3196–3204. Retrieved from: <https://www.ncbi.nlm.nih.gov/pubmed/26184647> https://doi.org/10.1093/cercor/bhv152

Perniss, P., Thompson, R. L., & Vigliocco, G. (2010). Iconicity as a general property of language: Evidence from spoken and signed languages. *Front. Psychol.*, 1, 227. Retrieved from: <https://www.ncbi.nlm.nih.gov/pubmed/21833282> https://doi.org/10.3389/fpsyg.2010.00227

Perniss, P., & Vigliocco, G. (2014). The bridge of iconicity: from a world of experience to the experience of language. *Philos. Trans. R Soc. Lond. B Biol. Sci.*, 369(1651), 20130300. Retrieved from: <https://www.ncbi.nlm.nih.gov/pubmed/25092668> https://doi.org/10.1098/rstb.2013.0300

Sacks, O. (1989). *Seeing voices: A journey into the world of the deaf*. Berkeley, CA: University of California Press.

Stamp, R., Schembri, A., Fenlon, J., Rentelis, R., Woll, B., & Cormier, K. (2014). Lexical variation and change in British Sign Language. *PLoS One* 9(4), e94053. Retrieved from: <https://www.ncbi.nlm.nih.gov/pubmed/24759673> https://doi.org/10.1371/journal.pone.0094053

Stokoe, W. C. (2005). Sign language structure: an outline of the visual communication systems of the American deaf. 1960. *J. Deaf. Stud. Deaf. Educ.*, 10(1), 3–37. Retrieved from: <https://www.ncbi.nlm.nih.gov/pubmed/15585746> https://doi.org/10.1093/deafed/eni001

Vinson, D. P., Cormier, K., Denmark, T., Schembri, A., & Vigliocco, G. (2008). The British Sign Language (BSL) norms for age of acquisition, familiarity, and iconicity. *Behav. Res. Methods* 40(4), 1079–1087. Retrieved from: <https://www.ncbi.nlm.nih.gov/pubmed/19001399> https://doi.org/10.3758/BRM.40.4.1079

Index